D0379842

SUGAR
FREE

SUGAR FREE

Karen Thomson
Introduction by Professor Tim Noakes

ROBINSON

ROBINSON

First published in Great Britain in 2016
by Robinson

Based on the South African version of
Sugar Free written by Karen Thomson
and Kerry Hammerton

Text copyright © Karen Thomson, 2016

Foreword for UK edition by
Dr Aseem Malhotra

Introduction by Professor Tim Noakes

Chapter Two: Understanding Sugar and
Carb Addiction by Dr Nicole Avena Ph.D.

Chapter Three: Getting Started on your
Sugar Free journey by Emily Maguire

Chapter Six: Low Carb Healthy Fat
Lifestyle by Emily Maguire

8 weeks of meal plans (vegetarian and
non-vegetarian) by Emily Maguire

3 5 7 9 8 6 4 2

The moral right of the authors has
been asserted.

All rights reserved.

No part of this publication may be
reproduced, stored in a retrieval system,
or transmitted, in any form, or by any
means, without the prior permission in
writing of the publisher, nor be otherwise
circulated in any form of binding or cover
other than that in which it is published
and without a similar condition including
this condition being imposed on the
subsequent purchaser.

Note The recommendations given in this
book are solely intended as education
and information and should not be
intended as medical advice.

A CIP catalogue record for this book is
available from the British Library.

ISBN: 978-1-47213-697-8 (paperback)

Designed by Andrew Barron,
thextension, and typeset in Adelle

Diagrams by Cedric Knight

Printed and bound in Great Britain
by Clays Ltd, St Ives plc

Papers used by Robinson are from
well-managed forests and other
responsible sources

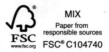

MIX
Paper from
responsible sources
FSC
www.fsc.org   FSC® C104740

Robinson
is an imprint of
Little, Brown Book Group
Carmelite House
50 Victoria Embankment
London EC4Y 0DZ

An Hachette UK Company

www.hachette.co.uk

www.littlebrown.co.uk

This book is dedicated to anyone who has ever struggled with their weight, body image or self esteem. You are worth so much more than you give yourself credit for.

'I saved the lives of 150 people through heart transplantations. If I had cared about preventative medicine earlier, I would have saved 150 million people.'

Professor Christiaan Barnard

Contents

Foreword

by **Dr Aseem Malhotra**

When Karen Thomson, the granddaughter of pioneering heart transplant surgeon Christiaan Barnard, invited me to speak at the world's first low-carb summit in South Africa in February 2015, the temptation was difficult to resist. Karen is courageously candid about her first-hand experience in overcoming addiction to alcohol and cocaine – and then to another 'pure, white and deadly' powder that has resulted in her opening the world's first carbohydrate and sugar-addiction rehab clinic, in Cape Town. When Karen told me that the event was being co-hosted by leading professor of exercise and sports medicine Tim Noakes, and that there was no food industry or pharmaceutical industry funding, any hesitation I had immediately disappeared. In the presentations that took place in late February, from a total of fifteen international speakers that included academic researchers and medical doctors, was an eloquent and evidence-based demolition job of current dietary guidelines that promote 'low fat' as best for weight and health. This convention will in my view go down in history as game-changing when it comes to dietary advice. And without Karen this summit would never have taken place.

But Karen is not just a health activist. She has utilised her passion and strong moral compass to address the single most important dietary factor that is contributing to a worldwide epidemic of obesity and type 2 diabetes: sugar. Don't get me wrong. Just as one cigarette won't kill you, neither will one teaspoon of sugar. But it's the consumption of sugar in excess over time that has the most devastating effect on our bodies. We are now witnessing the consequences on an epic scale, driven mainly by sugar in various forms being added to almost 80 per cent of all processed foods. As a result our sensitivity to sugar has gone down – and as any addict knows this leads to craving and consuming more and more.

To her credit, Karen was able to overcome her own addictions and realise the negative impact sugar was having on her health. Not only has Karen turned her life around, she has continued in the footsteps of her grandfather Christiaan Barnard and made a no less significant contribution to helping save lives by drawing on her own experiences. Rather than save people from drowning, it's better they're not thrown into the river in the first place. This book is a testament to a sugar-free enjoyment of food, life, health and happiness. Sugar is not evil in itself, but there's no doubt that life is a lot better without it.

Introduction

by **Professor
Tim Noakes**

Our lives are often directed by key moments, the importance of which we realise only years later. If ever.

On Sunday 3 December 1967, I was in Los Angeles, Southern California, the privileged recipient of a scholarship allowing me to study for one year at Huntington Park High School. At 3 p.m. that afternoon I was travelling back to Los Angeles after a visit to the Mission San Juan Capistrano. By chance, the radio was on. The 3 p.m. news started with a story that changed my life for ever. It began: 'A surgical team in Cape Town, South Africa, has performed the world's first successful human heart transplant.'

For a moment I was utterly stunned. How could this possibly be? Exposed as I was then to the magnitude of resources and world-leading sophistication of the United States in all matters, I naturally assumed that all world-changing events began in the United States. Later I learnt that the world's most experienced heart surgeons worked at Stanford University in California, a few hundred miles north of Los Angeles. It was expected that they would be the first to perform this miracle. How could surgeons from my small home town at the southern tip of the Darkest Continent have bested their efforts?

By the evening I knew more about the Cape Town surgical team: it was led by Professor Christiaan Barnard at the Groote Schuur Hospital with the involvement of the University of Cape Town. At the time I did not know that the recipient of this new heart, Louis Washkansky, was a diabetic whose heart had been irreparably damaged by his disease. Or that there is a body of strong scientific evidence linking sugar consumption to the development of type 2 diabetes.

Two weeks later Professor Barnard travelled to the United States to appear on *Face the Nation*, the most important US television programme of the day. I was utterly captivated. He seemed so young to have achieved such a remarkable breakthrough. He was unpretentious, sharp-witted and absolutely precise in his answers. His manner was full of dignity and calm, unintimidated by the media frenzy unleashed by the operation. He had a confidence and a presence I had rarely seen before, especially in someone so suddenly exposed to an intense global scrutiny. His TV appearance that day had a profound effect on my subconscious mind – one that eventually determined my future direction.

In time, Professor Barnard became the most famous doctor on the globe. And for good reason. He was one of South Africa's most remarkable men – a comparative genius who relished the challenge of going where no human in the long history of medicine had ventured. He played on the frontier between life and death. Professor Barnard and his team achieved the highest success rate for this operation in the world. Ultimately this was because he began with a vision and expressed the self-belief that his team was destined to achieve that vision. Later he reflected: 'Others believed in the work and soon came to labour through the night in a bare room ... They came, as I did, with the belief that we were going to find a medical truth. Being young, we did not question the origin of our belief. We had it, we felt it, and it was this which drove us on to its dramatic end.'

Precisely three months after that first operation, a short time before I was due to return to Cape Town, I awoke one morning with a message from my subconscious brain: 'Tim, when you return to Cape Town you will apply to study medicine at the University of Cape Town and will make medicine your profession.' Which is exactly what I did. And that is why each day I am grateful to Professor Barnard for giving me a direction in life that I might not otherwise have chosen.

The link to this book, of course, is that Karen Thomson is Professor Barnard's granddaughter. Karen is also the daughter of Deirdre Barnard, my contemporary, and a school friend of my wife Marilyn.

But it took life-changing events in both our lives for me to meet my icon's granddaughter.

On 12 December 2010, forty-three years and a few days after the first human heart transplant, I experienced the second epiphanic moment in my life. I decided that the way I had been eating for thirty-three years since I'd graduated as a medical doctor was harming my health, even though it was the approach prescribed by my profession. I decided to begin following a diet that was the polar opposite of what I had been taught was healthy. And so I removed almost all carbohydrates and all sugar from my diet and began to eat more protein and fat. The effect on my health was revolutionary. I went from feeling my age to suddenly feeling twenty years younger. My running responded in much the same way, so I was able to match the running times last recorded in my early forties.

For at least a year I hid my secret from all those who didn't see me in person and so were unaware of the very large weight loss consequent on my dietary change. Then Derek Watts interviewed me on *Carte Blanche*, South Africa's long-running investigative journalism programme, and cheekily asked me whether I would advise removing the thick layer of fat on the lamb chop he offered me for lunch. When I said we should eat the fat and throw away the meat, my story was suddenly out in the open. And not everyone was, or is, amused.

Karen Thomson was also watching that programme: her epiphanic moment came when she heard me say something to the effect that my eating plan removes hunger, whereas carbohydrates – and especially sugar – induce addictive-type eating behaviours. Working in the field of addiction treatment, her immediate response was: do people with other addictions also have addictive eating patterns? And, if so, might a sugar-free, low-carbohydrate, higher-fat diet help them overcome their primary addictions? And, if sugar addiction exists, might it not be possible to treat the condition according to the same principles used in the management of other addictions?

Karen's disposition towards asking these difficult questions to help patients struggling with complex health issues demonstrates that, like her grandfather, she has become a medical pioneer. Karen's vision led to developing the world's first programme devoted to managing sugar addiction according to established methods used for treating other addictions. She asks the question: is morbid obesity in some people really an unrecognised sugar addiction that can only be 'cured' if it is treated as an addiction of the same sort as heroin, cocaine and alcohol addictions?

The *Sugar Free* book describes Karen's personal and professional odyssey to this newfound vision. In taking this route she is blazing a new trail for the rest of the world to follow. When the messages in this book become fully understood, we will better appreciate the probable role of sugar addiction in the modern global epidemics of obesity and diabetes. For unless we understand exactly how sugar influences our appetites and food choices, it is unlikely we will ever be able to reverse those twin epidemics – the greatest challenges to human health ever.

It was said of Professor Barnard that his greatest desire was to help his patients improve their quality of life. Towards the end of his life he wrote that his personal surgical skills had helped hundreds of individual patients, but if he had devoted himself to the prevention of disease, he might have helped hundreds of millions more.

In writing this book, Karen Thomson is reaching out to those millions her grandfather did not reach. The extent to which sugar addiction impairs the health of the world's population is unknown, but it is likely to be a greater order of magnitude than we currently appreciate. Like the failed heart removed by Karen's grandfather's surgical scalpel, the scourge of sugar and its addiction must be excised from our society if we are to help those who are most vulnerable.

By bringing the topic into the open and exposing her personal journey, Karen Thomson is the pioneer and leader, driving us on to its dramatic end.

Karen's grandfather would be just so proud.

When to seek help

This book is a tool for self-exploration. All the suggestions made in the book are based on the author's personal experiences. If at any point in your own self-exploration you become overwhelmed by your feelings or think you cannot cope, please seek professional help.

If you feel in need of immediate assistance at any time, please contact an organisation such as the Samaritans. Find your local branch online or in the telephone directory. You could also talk to a professional therapist or psychologist.

This book should not be used to diagnose or test medical conditions. If you are at risk of any medical condition, please consult your GP before making any of the diet and lifestyle changes recommended in this book.

If you have any medical conditions such as hypothyroidism, diabetes, high blood pressure, high cholesterol or cardiac disease, I strongly recommend that you work with an integrative medical practitioner to help you manage your condition in a holistic manner.

Recommended professional resources

Online resource and support
The Sugar Free Revolution, thesugarfreerevolution.com
HELP: Harmony Eating & Lifestyle Program, helpdiet.co.za

Group support
Overeaters Anonymous, oa.org
Overeaters Anonymous Great Britain, oagb.org.uk

Health and exercise community
Smash the Fat, smashthefat.com

Ten guiding principles

1

Quit all sugar. One day at a time, with the support of the Sugar Free Revolution community, you can do this! Encourage, inspire and support each other on social media or find a partner or friend to do it with.

2

We dream BIG. We have a vision for ourselves and how we want our lives to be. We treat life as an adventure and don't settle for mediocrity. We do what we love and banish any potential 'what if' thoughts.

3

We give our bodies the foods they deserve. We understand that 'food is thy medicine' and the fuel our bodies need to perform daily activities. We think about what we put into our bodies and understand that you can't out-gym a bad diet.

4

We move our bodies. We perform some form of movement each day and love our bodies as the unique gifts they are. We believe in training smarter, not harder, and know that there is more to life than numbers on the scales, weights lifted or reps performed.

5

We see health as a lifestyle, not a quick fix. We are in this for the long haul and embrace the journey of a healthy body, mind and spirit rather than treating it as a destination. Similarly, we know that health is more just than abs and toned muscles.

6

We believe our thoughts create our reality. Our internal world shapes our external world. We realise that negative thoughts are easily replaceable with positive thoughts and we always strive to see the positive in any situation.

7

We surround ourselves with the right people. The people we spend the most time with play a huge role in our success. Further, we treat new people as friends we haven't met yet rather than strangers. You never know who's in the audience.

8

We express gratitude. Every day. We take time each day to be thankful for the things – no matter how big or small – and people in our lives.

9

We value experience over stuff. We know that happiness does not lie within material possessions, but rather in experiences that make us happy.

10

We know there is no such thing as failure. There is only learning. In the same way, the only 'bad' decision is not making a decision in the first place. It is better to act, observe and adjust than to be paralysed into indecision.

Sugar Free

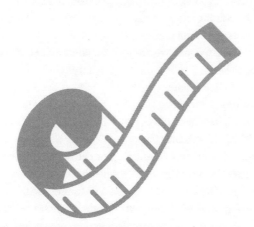

1   What is this book about?

The new food revolution has arrived. For decades, we have been urged to base our diets on carbohydrates and to restrict our intake of fats. This has resulted in a global epidemic of obesity-related diseases, and has led many people to become dependent on sugary and starchy foods. Today, an ever-increasing body of scientific evidence is showing the benefits of a new way of eating, based on low carbohydrates and healthy fats (LCHF).

Up until approximately 150 years ago sugar was not a staple in our diets. Fast-forward to today and we are consuming over 50 kilograms of sugar per year. This equates to about 29 teaspoons (both added and natural) every day, with 75 per cent of that from junk food and sugary drinks. Shocking, isn't it?

Lifestyle-related illnesses such as diabetes, metabolic syndrome, cardiovascular disease, insulin resistance, mood disorders, ADHD (attention deficit hyperactivity disorder), hyperactivity and certain types of cancers are skyrocketing. Our obesity epidemic is out of control and despite being told to 'eat less and exercise more' we are only getting sicker and fatter!

What if a single ingredient added to our food supply just over 100 years ago has wreaked havoc on our health? Is it possible that refined sugar – devoid of nutrients and high in calories – is causing our health to decline and our waistlines to expand? What if I told you that sugar is highly addictive, toxic and ruining your health? I absolutely am.

Luckily, the new food revolution has arrived. Everyone is talking about it, many are following it, and it's all about sugar-free living.

Numerous blogs and books can tell you how to cut sugar and refined carbohydrates out of your diet. Some are focused on family meals while others share great recipes and food ideas. Most provide diets and meal plans but fail to address the underlying emotional attachment you may have to sugar and carbs.

So what makes this book different?

I advocate the Low Carb Healthy Fat (LCHF) way of eating (see Chapter Three for what you can or can't eat, portion sizes and healthy food basics). But if you're a sugar and carb addict like me, then understanding what to eat and how much to eat is only half the story. Your relationship with food may be stuck in a destructive pattern. Perhaps you overindulge, comfort eat or binge. Perhaps sugar and carbs fill a greater void in your life than merely satisfying a physical craving.

The LCHF way of eating will help you beat your sugar and carb addiction, but you also need to examine your underlying thoughts, feelings and behaviours that are keeping you stuck in your unhealthy lifestyle. Cutting sugar is not a diet but a nutritional reset to enable you to break the cycle of sugar reliance and addiction.

Throughout this book I will focus on providing you with the tools and techniques you need to help you overcome addictive patterns and behaviours in your life as they relate to sugar and carb addiction. I have called on leading experts in the field of addiction and nutrition to provide you with cutting-edge science. Neuroscientist Dr Nicole Avena will explain exactly what sugar and carb addiction is and put you on the path to newfound food freedom while nutritionist Emily Maguire will explain the low-carb lifestyle devoid of deprivation and restriction.

My philosophy for the eight-week Sugar Free programme is based on five principles on which I base my own lifestyle

1
Cut out refined sugar and junk food.

2
No refined grains or processed vegetable oils.

3
Fat is your friend.

4
Great health starts in your kitchen; try to prepare as much of your own food as possible.

5
Empower yourself in body, mind and spirit.

✳
I truly want to help you become the healthy and amazing person you're meant to be.
✳
My Sugar Free eight-week programme will help you lay a strong foundation and guide you towards harmony, balance and health by empowering you in body, mind and spirit.
✳
I am with you every step of the way.

Who am I?

My name is Karen Thomson and I am a sugar and carb addict.
My love affair with sugar and carbohydrates – and loathing of myself and my body – started when I was four years old. I have starved, mutilated, gorged and disrespected myself in too many ways to mention. There had always been an underlying core belief that there was something intrinsically wrong with me that could only be fixed by the consumption of substances. My addictive cycle has led me to dependence on alcohol and cocaine and pretty much any substance or person that for a short space of time could make me feel good about myself. I have struggled with low self-esteem and low self-worth my entire life, always feeling that I was lacking in every way. I never felt beautiful, confident or adequate and I self-medicated these feelings with numerous substances and behaviours.

My alcohol and cocaine addiction brought me to my knees and forced me into an addiction treatment centre, but my spiritual rock bottom is what was truly driving my downward spiral. I slowly started to realise that there was no external solution for an internal problem and that to live a life in recovery I would have to restore myself to my natural way of being.

Stopping using drugs and alcohol was the easy part – but when my counsellor in treatment suggested that I had an eating disorder I balked at the idea. My great resistance to accepting this part of myself has in turn led to the greatest healing. I had to admit to myself and others just how destructive I had been. By examining the patterns in my past I came to realise that I suffered from a disease, the disease of addiction.

I had always sought relationships, work situations and events that reinforced my core belief: 'I am not valuable and will never be good enough.' From starting modelling at the age of sixteen to entering into abusive relationships, every path I chose and every person I had in my life clearly showed me that I deserved to be rejected, humiliated and used. I became a victim of my own choices.

'Why is this happening to me? It's just not fair,' was my overriding thought. I felt at the mercy of my circumstances and completely out of control. My only comfort was food. If I could not control my outside environment then I would control my body. Every let-down, angry and bad feeling I could not verbalise I took out on my body. I starved, binged and purged.

Shame, fear and guilt became permanent visitors in my life. I could not go on like this. I completed nine months in rehab and started on my life in recovery, but something was not right. I was still self-medicating, this time with something very acceptable and legal . . . I was feeding my feelings, whether happy or sad, with sugar and carbohydrates.

My dietitian in treatment had encouraged me to have cola, chocolate and other junk food in moderation. I complied and this was seen as a great success in the treatment of my eating disorder. The effects on my body and moods were not so great. I craved sugar; I needed sugar to survive. My daily cola (or three) had become my drug of choice. I soothed myself with this sweet, toxic liquid. My blood sugar would dip and I would turn into a monster: the sugar monster had arrived. I would be miserable, shaky and down until I could get my hands on my next sugar fix.

I realised I had a problem with sugar and carbohydrates after watching Professor Tim Noakes on a South African TV show. He mentioned the addictive nature of sugar and in that moment I knew that at the core of my being I had this problem. I was a sugar addict.

I examined my 'health-conscious, low-fat, restrictive diet' and realised that I was consuming just under forty teaspoons of sugar per day! The World Health Organisation (WHO) recommends four to nine teaspoons of sugar per day; I was consuming ten times that on a good day.

→

So what was I eating on an average day?

BREAKFAST

Coffee with two sugars

Low-fat bran and raisin muffin with margarine

Medium banana

LUNCH

Baked potato with fat-free cottage cheese

Salad with fat-free dressing

SNACK

Muesli bar with dried fruit

Cola

DINNER

Pasta with reduced-fat pasta sauce

Tea with two teaspoons of honey

I was always hungry, never satisfied and just plain miserable.

I started following a Low Carb Healthy Fat eating plan and the results were beyond my wildest expectations. I had to cut out sugar and refined carbohydrates completely. I was powerless over them: once I had one bite or sip I could not stop. The feelings of guilt and shame that came with the knowledge that 'Oh no, I have done it again' were just not worth it any more.

I lost weight, cellulite started disappearing and my appetite stabilised, but the greatest benefit by far was that my moods stabilised. I was no longer dependent on another substance to make me feel 'normal'. I was slowly restoring myself to my natural way of being.

Now who are you?

My story may seem extreme, but it wasn't until I started acknowledging my addiction to sugar and refined carbs that I was able to see just how bad it had become.

Now that you know a little bit about me, take some time to think about yourself and write down your own weight history. Later in the book I'll help you use this history for your recovery.

JOURNAL EXERCISE
Your weight history

The following ten questions will help you to write your own weight history.

1 Did you have weight issues as a child? What were your and your family's eating habits?
2 When did you first go on a diet and why? Was it your choice or someone else's?
3 When did you lose or gain weight? What happened in your life at the time?
4 Which successful diets have you tried (successful means you lost weight)?
5 Which unsuccessful diets have you tried (unsuccessful means you didn't lose and may have gained weight)?
6 Do you want to lose weight? If so, why?
7 How do you feel about yourself in general, and your body in particular, now?
8 What are your current eating habits? Do you eat three meals a day including breakfast? What do you snack on?
9 When and how do you eat 'forbidden' foods (the foods usually banned or limited in a diet, that you eat to help manage your feelings) such as chocolate, sugar, pasta and bread?
10 Do you ever lie about the amounts or types of foods you have eaten?

☎
Those questions may have brought up a lot of emotion for you. It's hard to admit that your eating is out of control. If at any time you feel you can't cope with these emotional feelings, please seek professional help.

15 ways to tell if you're a sugar and carb addict

You may have a problem with food, your weight or overeating, but are you actually addicted to sugar and carbs? There isn't a blood test that will tell you. It's something you have to figure out for yourself. I've put together a simple questionnaire to help you identify whether you may have a problem with your sugar and carb consumption. Be as honest as possible; ultimately, you are only accountable to yourself.

Do you

1
eat starchy or sweet, fatty foods until you feel uncomfortably full (bloated)?

2
feel hungry after eating a full meal even before it's time for your next meal?

3
eat large quantities of sweets or stodgy foods even though you aren't physically hungry?

4
feel self-loathing, disgust or depressed about your eating habits?

5
turn to carbohydrate-rich foods or sugar when feeling down or upset?

6
find you need more and more sweet foods to feel better?

7
plan to eat a small portion but end up binge eating?

8
find it difficult to cut back on starchy, sweet or fatty foods?

9
have a difficult time stopping, once you start eating starches, snack foods, junk food or sweets?

10
feel your eating habits are impacting negatively on your social, work or physical abilities?

11
find you cannot stick to healthy eating resolutions?

12
feel you need to (have to) have something sweet after lunch or dinner?

13
eat sweets and chocolates secretly and hide the wrappers because you don't want anyone to know?

14
eat one piece of cake and then come back for more and more?

15
feel as if you have a foggy head or your thoughts are unclear?

If you answered yes to at least five questions then you need to recognise you could be a sugar and carb addict.

You are not alone. I and hundreds of others who have completed my programmes identify as sugar and carb addicts, too. In fact many people out there would recognise themselves in these statements.

The Yale Food Addiction Scale (YFAS) is a more refined way of helping you determine if you are a food addict. Find a link to it at thesugarfreerevolution.com.

Karen

When I looked at this list of ways to tell if you are a sugar and carb addict, I realised I could identify with every one of those statements. When it comes to sugar and carbohydrates 'one is too many and a thousand never enough' – once sugar passes my lips I feel powerless to stop. I use sugar and carbs to comfort, soothe, reward and punish myself. The compulsion, obsessive thoughts and change in my behaviour are those of an addict in active addiction. When sugar hits my system it acts very similarly to other drugs I've used and the cravings are relentless. The hardest part of stopping is to remain stopped. My sugar withdrawals are intense and all-consuming; for me the term white-knuckling takes on new meaning.

Addiction is a disease that eats away at our freedom of choice and wellbeing, rendering us powerless over our 'drug of choice'. What makes admitting being addicted to sugar and carbs so hard is that it is socially acceptable and legal. If you are not yet convinced turn to Chapter Two, where neuroscientist Dr Nicole Avena explains exactly why she believes that sugar and carb addiction is real.

Here are some testimonials from some of the amazing people who have completed my programmes:

'This eight-week sugar and carb addiction programme helped me face my addictive patterns of functioning. Yes, I am an addict!'

'A great way to improve your health: it really works. I have lost 18kg in four months and my high blood sugar is a thing of the past.'

'It is changing my perspective on food. Also loving how I am learning to deal with real issues and not just being told what to eat.'

'Since reducing my intake of sugar – and I haven't even got around to the "hidden" sugars yet – there has been a significant decrease in my headaches and I no longer wake with a "foggy" head which persists for most of the day. No longer reaching for painkillers just to cope with a day's work. Have more energy, clarity of thought and more focus.'

'Sugar Free UK; lost 12.7kg in just over two and a half months. Enjoying the sugar- and carb-free existence, thanks to you. Miracle life change.'

'Well done Karen Thomson for believing in the addictive nature of sugar and continuing to fight for the cause and getting that message out there to the general public. I am a sugar addict. I can also not have one square of chocolate. I want the whole slab and another one and another one. Experts can tiptoe around the conceptualisation all they want, but if you are honest with yourself and if you have been down that road you know very well you don't care what it is called – you are eating to fill the void inside. This is what I did when my dad passed away; I tried soothing my heartache with chocolates and of course it didn't do the trick. My name is Zelda and I am a sugar addict. Spread the word – it is VERY real!'

'Just bought the book. Reading labels has been blowing my mind. I have years of avoiding fat to come to terms with but sugar is my real problem (insulin resistance).'

Throughout this book I will be sharing my personal journey with you. I will also introduce you to others who have managed to overcome their sugar and carb addiction, lose weight and embrace a new lifestyle in recovery by admitting that they were indeed slaves to sugar and carbs.

Admitting you are a sugar and carb addict may be hard, but living a life in recovery could give you a life beyond your wildest expectations.

Journalling your thoughts and feelings

As part of the preparation for your journey to recovery you'll need a journal or notebook where you can write down your reflections and answers to the exercises throughout this book. A simple notebook will do, or you may prefer one with an inspiring cover or message.

I've already asked you to write down answers to questions and will continue to encourage you to reflect on your feelings as part of the eight-week programme. On a weekly basis I'll also give you exercises and questions to help you reflect on your recovery process.

Why I wrote this book

I created the Harmony Eating & Lifestyle Program (HELP), according to my knowledge the only sugar and carbohydrate addiction inpatient treatment programme in the world, after I experienced the benefits and freedom of sugar-free eating in my own life. Too many people feed their feelings with sugar and carbs – the world's obesity problems clearly point in this direction. We are a society in turmoil, looking for external fixes to internal problems.

I truly believe we have everything we need within ourselves. Through working on the programme outlined in this book I've slowly been restoring my body, mind and spirit to its natural way of being. I have never experienced such freedom and joy. I've also witnessed it in so many others who have chosen to live a life in recovery from sugar and carbohydrate addiction.

My greatest realisation is that we are capable of far more than we give ourselves credit for. Today I am committed to myself and to my recovery. Life still happens but I'm now equipped with the tools to deal with it, without using drugs, alcohol, sugar or carbs. Recovery is a 'just for today' process that has to be taken one step at a time.

Through running HELP and seeing how people's lives have changed, I encourage you, in picking up this book, to commit to your authentic self. To acknowledge and accept who you really are, not who you think society or your parents want you to be. Today I love and accept myself exactly as I am; I hope that through following the suggestions in this book you will love and accept yourself, too.

2 Understanding sugar and carb addiction

'Sugar is eight times more addictive than cocaine. And what's interesting is that while cocaine and heroin activate only one spot for pleasure in the brain, sugar lights up the brain like a pinball machine!'
Dr Mark Hyman

Written with Nicole Avena Ph.D. and registered dietitian Kristen Criscitelli

What does it mean to be an addict?

Addiction is a multifaceted disorder caused by different factors, including biology, environment and culture.

According to the American Society of Addiction Medicine, addiction is defined as 'a primary, chronic disease of brain reward, motivation, memory and related circuitry.'[1] People can be addicted to and dependent on substances such as nicotine, heroin, cocaine or alcohol, and more recently, research has been emerging on the topic of behavioural addictions – such as sex. In fact, gambling was added to the most recent edition of the Diagnostic and Statistical Manual of Mental Disorders, which is considered the primary reference for mental health professionals.

At first, using a substance or engaging in a particular behaviour can be incredibly rewarding. But with continued use, a person may feel completely powerless over their need for the reward. An addict will compulsively pursue the reward despite the negative impact that it may have on interpersonal relationships, overall health and work. At this point the person can't voluntarily give up the behaviour, and is said to be in active addiction.

Addiction is chronic and progressive, which means the condition will always be present and that, without treatment, the symptoms get worse over time. To achieve and sustain recovery from addiction, abstinence from the addictive substance and/or behaviour, and daily maintenance by the addict, are required.

Our brain is comprised of different regions, and these regions communicate with each other by certain messenger chemicals, called neurotransmitters. External factors, as well as what is happening inside of our bodies, will influence the release of different neurotransmitters.

One neurotransmitter in particular that is released as a result of rewarding or pleasurable experiences – including sex, food intake and drug use – is dopamine. A characteristic shared by both addictive drugs and pleasurable

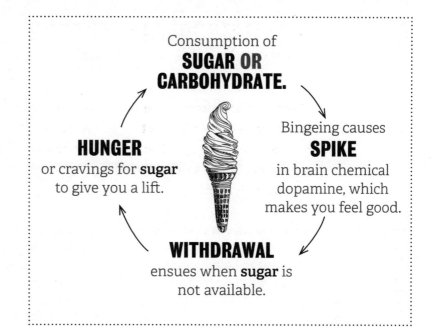

Consumption of
SUGAR OR CARBOHYDRATE.

HUNGER
or cravings for **sugar**
to give you a lift.

Bingeing causes
SPIKE
in brain chemical
dopamine, which
makes you feel good.

WITHDRAWAL
ensues when **sugar** is
not available.

experiences is the ability to increase dopamine levels and work within the regions of our brain associated with reward – and under certain circumstances, this same response is elicited with sugar. Dopamine is associated with reinforcement and addiction: it increases the likelihood that we will seek the pleasure and reward again and again.

Research in both animals and humans shows that sugar alters our brain's biochemical pathways, and studies have likened it to drugs typically involved in addiction.

Can sugar really be addictive?

Although the concept of sugar addiction has been around for many years, more and more studies are showing that it is indeed very plausible.

Several animal studies have found that sugar fulfils many of the criteria necessary to be considered to have addictive potential:[2]

1

Bingeing: Bingeing is defined as an escalation of intake and a period of excessive indulgence, which normally occurs after a period of abstinence or deprivation. Rats that have their sugar and chow (nutritionally balanced grain-based food) supply restricted intermittently will binge on sugar as soon as they're offered enough. Over time, the rats' sugar intake progressively increases.[3] This bingeing is accompanied by spikes of dopamine levels in their brains, a response that is associated with a pleasurable sensation. Notably, rats that have unlimited access to sugar and chow and do not binge on sugar do not show this same pattern of dopamine release.

2

Withdrawal: Following discontinuation of an addicting substance, withdrawal occurs, which is often painful and manifests both physically and psychologically. When the rats' sugar is taken away, they show signs of withdrawal. These signs include anxiety, aggression, teeth chattering and gnawing on the crate, as well as body shakes.[4]

3

Craving: Defined as an intense and powerful desire to obtain a substance of abuse, as a result of dependence or abstinence. After thirty days of enforced sugar abstinence, rats with a history of high sugar intake display a greater craving for sugar, as evidenced by the fact that they will work harder than before to receive it. This craving grows even stronger with longer abstinence.[5]

4

Cross-sensitisation: Research has shown that sugar-addicted rats more readily become addicted to other drugs of abuse, as well as alcohol.[6, 7, 8]

5

Use despite consequences: Unlike rats with chow, rats with access to a sugary food will continue to consume the sweet food even

when shown a cue that used to be accompanied by a mild electric shock, indicating compulsive eating that is not stopped by signals of potential negative effects.[9] Furthermore, rats with previous access to sugary food were more resistant to mild electric shock when compared to rats with previous access to methamphetamine.[10]

In other words, sugar can lead to patterns of behaviour that resemble those often associated with substance dependence.

Eating in response to our reward system

Our food intake is regulated by two drives, namely the homeostatic and hedonic pathways. Although the main drive for us to eat is to obtain the necessary energy (calories) and nutrients needed to sustain life, it is becoming increasingly evident that our food intake is closely intertwined with pleasure, emotions and reward.

The homeostatic pathway is a complex system that controls energy balance. Based on our nutritional state, hormones and peptides originating from our fat cells and our gastrointestinal tract signal our brain to stimulate intake or trigger feelings of satiety.[11, 12]

In contrast, the hedonic pathway has less to do with internal signalling of hunger and satiety and more to do with the pleasurable and motivating

CHAPTER TWO

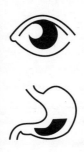

Eating for **SURVIVAL** the **homeostatic** pathway	Eating for **PLEASURE** the **hedonic** pathway
When the food reaches the stomach and intestines, chemical messengers slow down digestion and signal to the brain to stop eating. Seeing dessert is not as tempting.	Seeing highly palatable foods activates reward-associated areas of the brain even after eating in some people.

aspects of food. Eating is naturally reinforcing, since we need to eat in order to live, but the hedonic drive can override our metabolic need. The hedonic pathway mediates our 'liking' and 'wanting' of food and is associated with the dopamine system in the brain. It is activated by food and associated reward cues and contributes to feeding behaviour. [13, 14]

The pleasurable feelings we get when we eat sugar explain why we find ourselves eating ice cream and sweets after dinner even though we are full. In a world where highly palatable foods surround us, alterations in our homeostatic and hedonic systems can contribute to overeating and obesity and lead to further changes in our metabolic and reward pathways.

With ongoing consumption of sugar and starchy foods, our bodies adapt to the amount of sugar consumed, so our tolerance or threshold increases, which results in more of these foods being required to create the same effect – drug addicts and alcoholics experience the same cycle. What we're doing

is continually stimulating the neurochemical reward centres in the brain. The biological signals that control hunger and satiety become overwhelmed by this stimulation and our bodies (and brains) no longer understand the normal signals. If you are a sugar, carb or food addict, you may not experience an 'off switch' in response to eating, which tells you that you have satisfied your hunger. This explains why eating until you are satisfied may not work for addictive personalities, even on a LCHF diet, and why portion control is necessary.

There are differences (observed by using fMRI scans) between lean and obese individuals in their responses to high-calorie food cues in areas of the brain associated with reward and taste. [15] After consuming a meal, obese individuals show a greater response to high-calorie food cues when compared to lean individuals; [16] this may play a role in overeating behaviours in obese individuals.

Furthermore, certain individuals display addictive-like eating behaviours similar to those of drug addiction. The Yale Food Addiction Scale (YFAS) is a validated scale that is used to identify feeding behaviours that are associated with addiction.[17] Higher scores on the YFAS are seen in people with type 2 diabetes and binge eating disorder as well as overweight and obese individuals.[18, 19]

Moreover, the types of food that are associated with addictive-like behaviours are highly processed and high in refined carbohydrates and sugar. These foods are changed from their natural state and have a high glycemic load (GL) – meaning they get absorbed quickly and cause a surge in blood sugar after being consumed. This may explain their addictive potential (though some industrially processed foods such as soya mince are low GL). Similarly, drugs of abuse are also changed from their natural state and absorbed quickly (think coca leaf being processed into cocaine). Recently, research showed that people with elevated YFAS scores (increased symptoms of addictive-like eating) report foods with high GL to be very problematic.[20]

Additionally, we believe sugar addiction also involves a compulsive pursuit of foods rich in sugar and carbohydrates in response to both positive and negative feelings. High-carbohydrate foods are great at raising levels of serotonin, which is a neurotransmitter associated with mood and happiness. This may explain why some of us – particularly those who struggle with carbohydrate cravings – turn to these types of foods when we're feeling down.

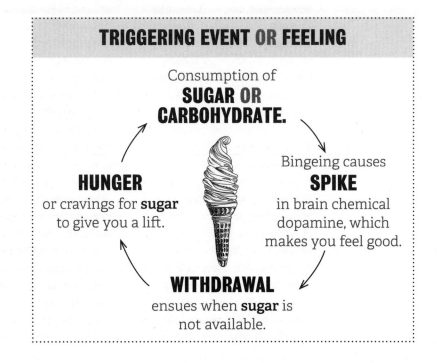

TRIGGERING EVENT OR FEELING

Consumption of
SUGAR OR CARBOHYDRATE.

Bingeing causes **SPIKE** in brain chemical dopamine, which makes you feel good.

WITHDRAWAL ensues when **sugar** is not available.

HUNGER or cravings for **sugar** to give you a lift.

CHAPTER TWO

Besides 'emotional eating', people may reach for highly palatable foods during times of stress. A recent study found that women who consumed sugar-sweetened beverages reduced the secretion of stress-induced cortisol (a hormone associated with stress) during an intentionally challenging mental arithmetic task. This helps explain why some people find themselves eating sugary foods to cope with problems. [21]

These highly palatable sugar-laden foods have not always been considered a significant problem in overriding our homeostatic drives. In the past, foods were seldom likened to drugs of abuse, but it is important to remember that our food landscape has undergone dramatic changes. About two hundred years ago, people in developed countries consumed approximately three kilograms of sugar per year; today our sugar intake exceeds 50 kilograms per year. [22]

The changing food environment

Our paleolithic ancestors were hunters and gatherers who had to forage and hunt for the food that they were going to consume, and so their energy intake (calories) closely matched their energy expenditure. However, since the beginning of the twentieth century, due to advances in technology, urbanisation and motorisation, the amount of calories needed on a daily basis has declined. At the same time, calorically dense, highly palatable foods were becoming more easily accessible and cheaper to obtain. Starting from the 1970s, refined carbohydrates and fats inundated the food supply, which increased the amount of available calories. [23]

On a daily basis the average person now eats about 22 teaspoons of added sugar, which equates to about 350 additional calories every day. No wonder obesity is such a problem!

It only takes a second to realise that the modern day 'obesogenic environment', in which people eat unhealthily and do not do enough exercise, is difficult to get away from. Highly palatable combinations of ingredients are omnipresent and you do not need to try very hard to get whatever you're craving at that exact moment.

Conversely, if you're trying to steer clear of sugar it may prove to be a difficult task since there are more than sixty different names it can go by. It easily sneaks into our foods as syrup, malt, agave nectar, caramel, beet sugar, apple juice from concentrate, honey and molasses. Other culprits include words ending in '-ose', such as dextrose, fructose, lactose, glucose and maltose. [24, 25] It is especially easy to be fooled when the word 'fruit' is used, suggesting that it is actually healthy, [26] but in reality these are all just different ways of saying the same thing – sugar!

BUTTERED SYRUP
CANE SUGAR CORN
Caramel SYRUP
Beet Sugar CANE JUICE
DEXTROSE
TREACLE Confectioner's Sugar
AGAVE NECTAR
Maltodextrin CAROB SYRUP
FRUCTOSE
DEHYDRATED CANE JUICE
Demerara Sugar
FRUIT JUICE RAW
CONCENTRATE SUGAR
Diastic Diatase MALT
MALTOSE MALT SUGAR
Molasses MANITOL
SUCROSE
SORGHUM SYRUP
Sorbitol CASTER SUGAR
YELLOW SUGAR
LACTOSE GRAPE SUGAR
GLUCOSE SOLIDS
BARLEY MALT
Golden Sugar Grape Sugar
REFINER'S SYRUP
GLUCOSE
DATE SUGAR
DEXTRAN FRUIT JUICE
MAPLE SYRUP
HONEY ICING SUGAR
HFCS HIGH FRUCTOSE CORN SYRUP

Too much sugar makes you ill

Sugar is now seen as potentially the central offender behind the rising global rates of obesity and a plethora of related disorders.

Children who consume more sugar and sugar-sweetened beverages are at increased risk of developing dental caries. [27]

People who consume more sugar-sweetened beverages and refined grains have been shown to be at increased risk of developing type 2 diabetes. [28] As sugar becomes more readily available around the world, the risk of diabetes prevalence increases. [29] Interestingly, recent research also shows that fructose (a naturally occurring sugar found in fruits, some vegetables, and honey, and a component of high fructose corn syrup) may also increase your risk for diabetes all on its own by raising blood sugar and insulin levels, while promoting insulin resistance. [30]

Sugar also contributes to the development of metabolic syndrome and heart disease. [31, 32] Excess sugar raises cholesterol levels, triglycerides, and blood vessel-clogging low-density lipoprotein (LDL) particles, as well as increasing the risk of high blood pressure (hypertension). [33]

Traditional wisdom claims that sugar contributes only 'empty' calories that are devoid of beneficial and filling nutrients – meaning that it's easy to overindulge on sugar without feeling satisfied. There is also compelling evidence showing that eating and drinking sugar increases your risk for developing obesity.[34, 35] Recent research also suggests that fructose may actually switch on fat production and storage and increase those particularly dangerous belly fat deposits.[36]

Too much sugar has a negative effect on cognition[37] and may be a risk factor for depression.[38] It also contributes to an inflammatory state within the body[39, 40] which may result in diseases such as osteoarthritis, dermatitis, psoriasis, various intestinal disorders and certain types of heart disease.

Overall, it is obvious that sugar's contribution to chronic disease and obesity is far more sinister than just being 'empty calories' as once thought.[41] The evidence is strong – we need not wait for more proof of sugar's detrimental effects before cutting our consumption. However, we wouldn't be in the midst of a global epidemic if it were that simple. The truth is, sugar can be a difficult addiction to break.

Ready to kick the sugar habit for good? In the next chapter we will give you the tools to help you get started.

REFERENCES

1 Definition of Addiction 2011 [cited 2015 July 29, 2015. Available from: http://www.asam.org/for-the-public/definition-of-addiction.

2 Avena, N.M., Rada, P. and Hoebel, B.G. Evidence for sugar addiction: behavioral and neurochemical effects of intermittent, excessive sugar intake. Neurosci Biobehav Rev, 2008. 32(1): p. 20–39.

3 Avena, N.M., Rada, P. and Hoebel, B.G. Daily bingeing on sugar repeatedly releases dopamine in the accumbens shell. Neuroscience, 2005. 134(3): p. 737–44.

4 Wideman, C.H., Nadzam, G.R., and Murphy, H.M. Implications of an animal model of sugar addiction, withdrawal and relapse for human health. Nutr Neurosci, 2005. 8(5–6): p. 269–76.

5 Grimm, J.W., Fyall, A.M., and Osincup, D.P. Incubation of sucrose craving: effects of reduced training and sucrose pre-loading. Physiol Behav, 2005. 84(1): p. 73–9.

6 Avena, N.M., et al., Sugar-dependent rats show enhanced intake of unsweetened ethanol. Alcohol, 2004. 34(2–3): p. 203–9.

7 Avena, N.M., and Hoebel, B.G. A diet promoting sugar dependency causes behavioral cross-sensitization to a low dose of amphetamine. Neuroscience, 2003. 122(1): p. 17–20.

8 Rorabaugh, J.M., Stratford, J.M., and Zahniser, N.R. Differences in bingeing behavior and cocaine reward following intermittent access to sucrose, glucose or fructose solutions. Neuroscience, 2015. 301: p. 213–220.

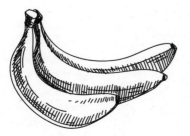

9   Velazquez-Sanchez, C., et al., Seeking behavior, place conditioning, and resistance to conditioned suppression of feeding in rats intermittently exposed to palatable food. Behav Neurosci, 2015. 129(2): p. 219–24.

10   Krasnova, I.N., et al., Incubation of methamphetamine and palatable food craving after punishment-induced abstinence. Neuropsychopharmacology, 2014. 39(8): p. 2008–16.

11   Tulloch, A.J., et al., Neural responses to macronutrients: hedonic and homeostatic mechanisms. Gastroenterology, 2015. 148(6): p. 1205–18.

12   Camilleri, M., Peripheral mechanisms in appetite regulation. Gastroenterology, 2015. 148(6): p. 1219–33.

13   Volkow, N.D., et al., Obesity and addiction: neurobiological overlaps. Obes Rev, 2013. 14(1): p. 2–18.

14   Yu, Y.H., et al., Metabolic vs. hedonic obesity: a conceptual distinction and its clinical implications. Obes Rev, 2015. 16(3): p. 234–47.

15   Pursey, K.M., et al., Neural responses to visual food cues according to weight status: a systematic review of functional magnetic resonance imaging studies. Front Nutr, 2014. 1: p. 7.

16   Dimitropoulos, A., et al., Greater corticolimbic activation to high-calorie food cues after eating in obese vs. normal-weight adults. Appetite, 2012. 58(1): p. 303–12.

17   Gearhardt, A.N., Corbin, W.R., and Brownell, K.D. Preliminary validation of the Yale Food Addiction Scale. Appetite, 2009. 52(2): p. 430–6.

18   Gearhardt, A.N., et al., An examination of the food addiction construct in obese patients with binge eating disorder. Int J Eat Disord, 2012. 45(5): p. 657–63.

19   Raymond, K.L., and Lovell, G.P. Food addiction symptomology, impulsivity, mood, and body mass index in people with type two diabetes. Appetite, 2015.

20   Schulte, E.M., Avena, N.M., and Gearhardt, A.N. Which foods may be addictive? The roles of processing, fat content, and glycemic load. PLoS One, 2015. 10(2): p. e0117959.

21   Tryon, M.S., et al., Excessive Sugar consumption may be a difficult habit to break: A view from the brain and body. J Clin Endocrinol Metab, 2015. 100(6): p. 2239–47.

22   Zuker, C.S., Food for the brain. Cell, 2015. 161(1): p. 9–11.

23   Swinburn, B.A., et al., The global obesity pandemic: shaped by global drivers and local environments. The Lancet, 2011. 378(9793): p. 804–814.

24   Frequently Asked Questions about Sugar. Getting Healthy [Webpage] 2014 May 19, 2014 [cited 2015 June 17, 2015]. Available from: http://www.heart.org/HEARTORG/GettingHealthy/NutritionCenter/HealthyDietGoals/Frequently-Asked-Questions-About-Sugar_UCM_306725_Article.jsp.

25   Empty Calories – Where are Added Sugars? [cited 2015 June 17, 2015]. Available from: http://www.choosemyplate.gov/weight-management-calories/calories/added-sugars.html.

26   Sutterlin, B., and Siegrist, M. Simply adding the word 'fruit' makes sugar healthier: The misleading effect of symbolic information on the perceived healthiness of food. Appetite, 2015. 95: p. 252–261.

27   Costacurta, M., et al., Dental caries and childhood obesity: analysis of food intakes, lifestyle. Eur J Paediatr Dent, 2014. 15(4): p. 343–8.

28   Schulze, M.B., et al., Dietary pattern, inflammation, and incidence of type 2 diabetes in women. Am J Clin Nutr, 2005. 82(3): p. 675-84; quiz 714–5.

29 Basu, S., et al., The relationship of sugar to population-level diabetes prevalence: an econometric analysis of repeated cross-sectional data. PLoS One, 2013. 8(2): p. e57873.

30 Khitan, Z., and Kim, D.H. Fructose: a key factor in the development of metabolic syndrome and hypertension. J Nutr Metab, 2013. 2013: p. 682673.

31 Dhurandhar, N.V., and Thomas, D. The link between dietary sugar intake and cardiovascular disease mortality: an unresolved question. Jama, 2015. 313(9): p. 959–60.

32 Malik, V.S., et al., Sugar-sweetened beverages and risk of metabolic syndrome and type 2 diabetes: a meta-analysis. Diabetes Care, 2010. 33(11): p. 2477–83.

33 Te Morenga, L.A., et al., Dietary sugars and cardiometabolic risk: systematic review and meta-analyses of randomized controlled trials of the effects on blood pressure and lipids. Am J Clin Nutr, 2014. 100(1): p. 65–79.

34 Hu, F.B., Resolved: there is sufficient scientific evidence that decreasing sugar-sweetened beverage consumption will reduce the prevalence of obesity and obesity-related diseases. Obes Rev, 2013. 14(8): p. 606–19.

35 Te Morenga, L., Mallard, S., and Mann, J. Dietary sugars and body weight: systematic review and meta-analyses of randomised controlled trials and cohort studies. BMJ, 2013. 346: p. e7492.

36 Stanhope, K.L., et al., Consuming fructose-sweetened, not glucose-sweetened, beverages increases visceral adiposity and lipids and decreases insulin sensitivity in overweight/obese humans. J Clin Invest, 2009. 119(5): p. 1322–34.

37 Micha, R., Rogers, P.J., and Nelson, M. Glycaemic index and glycaemic load of breakfast predict cognitive function and mood in school children: a randomised controlled trial. Br J Nutr, 2011. 106(10): p. 1552–61.

38 Gangwisch, J.E., et al., High glycemic index diet as a risk factor for depression: analyses from the Women's Health Initiative. Am J Clin Nutr, 2015.

39 Aeberli, I., et al., Low to moderate sugar-sweetened beverage consumption impairs glucose and lipid metabolism and promotes inflammation in healthy young men: a randomized controlled trial. Am J Clin Nutr, 2011. 94(2): p. 479–85.

40 Benetti, E., et al., High sugar intake and development of skeletal muscle insulin resistance and inflammation in mice: a protective role for PPAR- delta agonism. Mediators Inflamm, 2013. 2013: p. 509502.

41 Singh, G.M., et al., Estimated Global, Regional, and National Disease Burdens Related to Sugar-Sweetened Beverage Consumption in 2010. Circulation, 2015.

3 Getting started on your Sugar Free journey

To help you get started we've put together a quick guide to the Low Carb Healthy Fat (LCHF) way of eating. These are the guiding principles around foods you can eat and those you should be avoiding.

Written with nutritionist Emily Maguire

A LCHF diet means you eat fewer carbohydrates and a higher portion of fat than you're used to. You also cut out sugar and starches (such as whole grains, cereals, bread, pasta, rice and potatoes). Many people mistake this diet for a high-protein diet. Yet, if followed correctly, fats instead of protein should replace carbohydrates – your protein consumption should remain similar to before.

If you research LCHF on the internet or in other books you'll find advice such as: eat until you're satisfied, you don't need to calorie count, you don't need to weigh your food. This is great advice – if you know when your body is telling you it's full and you're able to listen. But as sugar and carb addicts we've overridden our body's natural satiety signals – we need to re-teach ourselves to listen to these.

What can you eat?

For the first eight weeks we're going to encourage you to exercise portion control and to measure certain foods such as proteins, fats and 'dense' vegetables. You can eat meat, fish, eggs, dairy products, vegetables (particularly those that grow above the ground), natural fats and some fruit.

People who have been used to having carbohydrates as the main staple of their diet may wonder how this is going to work, but there truly is an abundance of amazing foods that you can eat. Let's begin by looking at these in terms of the three main food groups, or macronutrients: protein, carbohydrates and fats.

THE LCHF FOOD PYRAMID

Healthy fats

Fruit, nuts and seeds

Dairy products, eggs and vegetables

Meat, poultry, and fish

Healthy fat and oils

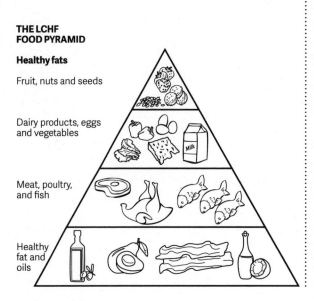

Karen

When I first started following the LCHF way of life I was thrilled that I could have eggs and bacon for breakfast, a huge salad with avocado, feta and nuts for lunch, and a steak with creamed spinach and extra butter for dinner. I'd listened to the experts on how to follow a low-carb high-fat meal plan and took their advice very seriously. When they said 'eat fat until you are stuffed' I truly took their advice to heart. I ate and ate and loved every minute. Apart from adding butter and cream to absolutely everything, I also upped my protein intake to absurd amounts, forgetting that this was a high-fat, not high-protein, eating plan.

I spent my day either eating, preparing to eat or thinking about what I was going to eat next. You see, even though I was abstinent from sugar I was overeating fat. So, no surprise, I ended up putting on weight. What had conveniently slipped my mind was that these experts were not addicts themselves, and as such were able to identify when they were full. I, on the other hand, can eat and eat and then eat some more without realising my body does not need more food. The part of my brain that is supposed to tell me I'm full and should stop eating just wasn't working.

I finally decided that despite the benefits I was experiencing from LCHF, my steadily increasing weight gain was not benefiting me. I needed professional help from someone who understood this way of eating.

Even though the LCHF way of eating is not about calorie counting, portion control is important. I went to see a dietitian who assisted me with portion sizes and meal planning. I realised I'd been eating about four times what I needed to consume daily.

PROTEIN

Meat, poultry and fish

An LCHF diet isn't excessively high in protein and generally you will find your portion sizes of these foods won't change too much from what you're having now. You can enjoy all forms of meat (including offal), poultry, game and fish and the fats that come with these foods, such as chicken skin and the fat on a juicy steak.

Eggs

These are in a category of their own because they are just an amazing staple in an LCHF diet. They are versatile, cheap and exceptionally nutritious. It used to be believed that eating more than two or three eggs per week would increase your risk of heart disease by raising your cholesterol level. However, it has now been found that the cholesterol that is contained within eggs does not raise your blood cholesterol level. Having a couple of eggs per day could actually have a positive effect on your health.

Dairy

Certain dairy options such as full-fat cream, cheeses, butter and whole-milk natural yogurt are all great to have as part of an LCHF diet. Whole milk in limited quantities can be OK but it has a high level of milk sugars (lactose). Although these sugars are naturally occurring, they are still sugar, so it is better to use cream in place of milk. Stick to one to two portions of dairy per day: a matchbox-sized piece of hard cheese or 250ml cream or whole-milk natural yogurt.

CARBOHYDRATES

Vegetables

The vegetables you eat will play a big part in where you get your carbohydrates. The majority of your meals will always include some form of vegetable, and it's a good idea to choose a variety of different vegetables, to ensure that you benefit from all of the vitamins, minerals and other beneficial compounds (phytochemicals) that they offer.

However, we suggest you limit your intake of certain vegetables, which we term 'dense' vegetables, because they contain higher proportions of starches and natural sugars. These include root vegetables such as beetroot, carrots, parsnips, turnips and sweet potatoes, butternut squash, pumpkin, sweetcorn, peas, beans and pulses (legumes) such as lentils, dried beans and chickpeas.

Quinoa is also allowed in limited quantities; it's an exception to our 'no grain' rule because the nutritional composition of quinoa is far lower in carbohydrates than other grains.

Limit these dense veg to ½ cup of the cooked or prepared veg per day – if you haven't got a standard cup measure, think of ½ cup as the size of a tennis ball.

Fruits

When you think of it fruits are generally sweet, yet they are often promoted in weight-loss programmes as OK to consume in abundance. The sweetness comes from two sugars, glucose and fructose, and although they are naturally occurring they are nonetheless sugars. That being said, some fruits are lower in sugar than others; berries are a good example. When eating higher-sugar fruits such as mangoes, melons, pineapple and stone fruit such as peaches it is recommended to have them along with some type of fat, such as cream, yogurt or nut butter.

Avoid grapes and bananas, dried and tinned fruits. When fruit juices and smoothies are processed the fibre is removed and so you are effectively consuming sugar in liquid form, which is why we advise you to choose any alternative drink.

FATS

Coconut oil, olive oil, olives, avocados, butter, ghee, nuts and seeds and nut butters will be staples of your LCHF diet: they are all healthy fats that can be added to your foods or used in recipes. You will also be eating fats that are found naturally in foods, such as cream and the fat on meats (bacon fat and duck, goose or chicken fat can be used for cooking, in addition to coconut oil and butter).

DRINKS

Water, both still and sparkling, is your best choice of drink. Add fresh lemon or lime for flavour. A good way to flavour a jug of water is to add some cut-up fruit and leave in the fridge overnight.

All tea (including breakfast, Earl Grey, herbal and fruit teas) and coffee are allowed. If you normally have sugar in your tea or coffee try replacing this with some cream with cinnamon.

What can't you eat?

As this will be a huge change in dietary lifestyle for many of you it's better to be 100 per cent sure as to what is off the menu. Generally all sugar, grains and processed oils need to be avoided.

SUGAR

It's not as simple as the white stuff you add to coffee and tea, and which makes sweet treats such as cakes and biscuits so irresistible to sugar and carb addicts. Sugar has over fifty different names, which the food industry has taken note of and uses to disguise the fact that sugar is hidden in a huge number of processed foods – both conventionally sweet and savoury. As well as table sugar, you'll avoid honey, maple syrup, treacle, molasses and agave nectar. You'll also stay away from cakes, pastries, muffins, biscuits and sweets, fizzy drinks (including sports drinks), fruit juices, sauces, jams and spreads, ice cream, sweetened yogurt and breakfast cereal (we'll show you how to make a nutritious nut granola).

STARCHY CARBOHYDRATES

Bread, pasta, rice and white potatoes are all too high in starchy carbohydrates for a LCHF lifestyle. And yes, we mean all types of bread, pasta (even wholewheat), rice, all types of wheat, oats, rye and barley.

PROCESSED OILS

Vegetable oils were once thought to be a healthy choice, but studies now show that these highly processed oils can be harmful to your health. Margarine is one of the worst offenders. Avoid all vegetable and seed oils – corn, sunflower, safflower, canola, rapeseed (often sold as 'vegetable oil') and soya/soybean oil – as well as margarine. For cooking, use heat-stable fats such as butter or coconut oil and for dressings use extra virgin olive oil

Sugar by any other name

Keep a look out for hidden sugar in the food you buy. It's often *disguised* under another name. See page 18 for a list of the numerous ways sugar can sneak into your diet.

FOODS TO AVOID

Sugar	Refined grains	Processed oils
Under any name (see page 18)	Bread	Canola oil
Honey	Pasta	Rapeseed oil
Cakes	Rice	Corn oil
Sweets	Pastries	Sunflower oil
Milk chocolate, white chocolate	Pies	Safflower oil
Jams	Breakfast cereals	Soybean oil
Marmalade	Cereal bars	Margarine
Syrup	Muffins	
Coconut sugar	Granola	
Agave nectar	Noodles	
Fruit juices		
Smoothies (unless our recipes)	White potatoes	
Canned fruit	Crisps (chips)	
Dried fruits		
Raisins		
Sweeteners		
Diet drinks		
Soft/fizzy drinks		
Vitamin or sports drinks		
Low-fat yogurts		
Fruit flavour yogurts		
Packaged sauces		

ALCOHOL: YOUR BEST CHOICES

Low-sugar alcohol	Higher-sugar alcohol
1 glass of red wine	All cocktails
1 glass of dry white wine	Rosé wine
1 glass of brut sparkling wine – cava, Prosecco, champagne	Sherry (both sweet and dry)
1 measure of vodka	Dark liquor – Jack Daniels, Southern Comfort etc
1 measure of gin	Cream liqueurs
1 measure of tequila	Cider
1 measure of whisky	Beer (regular)
Low-sugar mixers – soda water, slimline tonic	Alcopops
1 small glass light beer	

Grey area: foods to limit

Freeing yourself from sugar and carb addiction and following a Low Carb Healthy Fat way of eating is a lifestyle change. If you are also using the eight-week programme in this book to help you lose weight, we advise against consuming alcohol or chocolate – at least until you have achieved your goal. However, we understand that finding balance is also important, to make sure you can stick with this for the long term.

ALCOHOL

As part of an LCHF lifestyle the best choices would be: 1 glass of red wine, dry white wine or sparkling wine (brut cava or champagne), 1 measure of vodka or gin with a low-sugar mixer (such as soda water or slimline tonic), 1 small glass of light beer. Look for beers with a total carb content of less than 2 per cent – you may have to look online because alcohol is not labelled with nutrition information.

Alcohol to be avoided includes regular beer, cider, rosé wine and any fruit- or cream-based cocktails.

DARK CHOCOLATE

The great thing about LCHF is that you can have chocolate. But it must have a high cocoa content: at least 70% and the higher the better. Have no more than two squares per day.

SWEETENERS

The first goal of the LCHF lifestyle is to get you free of sugars and refined grains. For many people the addiction to sugar can be so great that using sweeteners as a tool may be necessary at first. That being said, keeping sweeteners in your diet can 'feed' your sweet tooth and spark sugar and carb cravings. In the first few weeks you may feel you need a natural sweetener such as stevia in your coffee or tea. If, however, after two or three weeks on your LCHF programme you are still feeling hungry or having sugar cravings then it could be due to the sweeteners. Try to gradually reduce the amount that you are using.

How much should you eat every day?
Although this way of eating is not about calorie counting, the Low Carb Healthy Fat lifestyle will not be healthy if you continually consume excess calories – particularly if you are trying to lose weight. Most women should be consuming between 1500 and 2000 calories (kcal) a day, and men between 2000 and 2500 calories. The exact intake will vary from person to person, depending on build, age and activity level; it can also vary from day to day.

PORTION SIZES
In this book, our portions equate to 1500 – 2000 calories a day. You will need to learn to exercise some discretion as to what is an appropriate portion for your gender, level of daily activity, desired outcome from following the sugar-free programme etc: older, less active, smaller-framed individuals and females should have smaller portions than younger, fitter, larger-framed males. Some people find that stopping when they're full is a useful indicator of how many portions

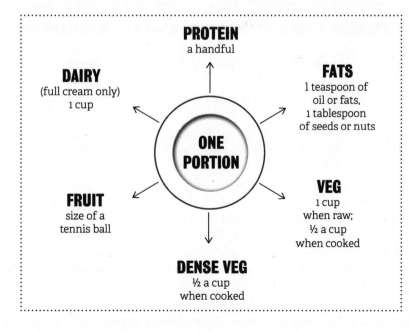

PROTEIN
a handful

DAIRY
(full cream only)
1 cup

FATS
1 teaspoon of
oil or fats,
1 tablespoon
of seeds or nuts

ONE PORTION

FRUIT
size of a
tennis ball

VEG
1 cup
when raw;
½ a cup
when cooked

DENSE VEG
½ a cup
when cooked

they should eat. If you don't feel comfortable judging when you're full, choose a medium range of portion size.

Try filling your plate as shown:

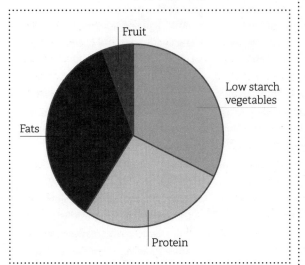

Fruit

Low starch vegetables

Fats

Protein

Eating principles

The eight-week plan includes three meals a day as well as snacks: this is a good starting template as you rid yourself of cravings. For many people this is a good way to continue on the LCHF lifestyle. But the great thing about LCHF and removing refined carbs from your diet is that you will be able to truly listen to your body again. You may find that you are not really hungry, and eating twice a day with one small snack suits you just fine. As long as you are listening to your body and nourishing it when it needs it, you are well on the way to living the LCHF lifestyle.

FAT IS YOUR FRIEND
The LCHF lifestyle emphasises the consumption of a higher amount

of healthy fats than you may be used to. This dietary change is probably the one that many people find the hardest. Just remember that a higher fat intake will keep you feeling fuller for longer and really will propel you closer to your goal of breaking your carb addiction and losing weight.

You will need to avoid most products that are labelled low-fat, fat-free or light, because these products often contain added sugar or sweeteners. Likewise, shop-bought products like mayonnaise will contain a lot of seed and vegetable oils. We have provided a mayonnaise recipe in the book so you can still enjoy a wide range of dishes with this versatile condiment.

LCHF and vegetarians

A vegetarian LCHF lifestyle can be achieved – though it may need a little more planning than for people who eat meat and fish. Your overall carbohydrate intake may also be slightly higher. To help you, we have included vegetarian meal plans for the eight-week programme.

If you are vegetarian, it is important to make sure that you are getting all of the vitamins and minerals that your body needs. As there are several nutrients, such as vitamin B12, that can only be found in animal products, it would be advisable to take a daily multivitamin tablet.

PROTEIN

While your sources of carbohydrates and fats will be exactly the same as for non-vegetarians, it is true that the proteins contained within animal products have greater bioavailability, which means that the body finds it easier to extract the nutrients that it needs. As long as you eat eggs and a good array of dairy products such as cheeses, cream and yogurt, your body will receive the nutrients that it needs.

Other protein sources in a vegetarian LCHF plan include pulses such as beans, lentils and chickpeas, and ancient grains such as quinoa. However, these are all fairly high in carbohydrates, so you need to be very careful on portion sizes. Nuts and seeds are good sources of protein as well as fat – but they are also high in carbohydrates when eaten in excess. A vegetarian protein powder that has 1g or less of sugar per 100g could be a useful addition to your diet.

LCHF and being dairy-free

If you don't eat dairy, you can swap each dairy portion for one of protein or fat, and add an additional portion of green leafy vegetables, such as spinach, broccoli and pak choi. Instead of one cup of cow's milk, you can drink a third of a cup of coconut milk, or one and a half to two cups of unsweetened almond milk. Remember to include other calcium-rich foods such as sardines, rhubarb, oranges, almonds and dark green leafy vegetables like kale.

Adjustments for those on medications

If you are on any form of medication it is advisable to check with your doctor before you start your LCHF journey. Once you are following this dietary approach, there are a few medications that will need to be monitored and adjusted.

Blood pressure medication One of the consistent findings with an LCHF diet is its ability to naturally lower the body's blood pressure. For individuals who are on blood pressure medications it is important to keep an eye on your blood pressure reading. Your medications may need to be reduced even within the first two weeks. Consult your GP before reducing any medication.

Diabetic medication The role of diabetic medications is to help the body to metabolise glucose in order to prevent high blood sugar levels. When you eat carbohydrates you raise your blood sugar level; diabetics need to take insulin to cope with this. As an LCHF diet has no sugars or grains and a low overall carbohydrate level, the need for insulin is greatly reduced. Make sure you measure your blood sugar levels at regular intervals throughout the day when you first start on this journey. If you are taking any form of fast-acting insulin, this may need to be stopped right away. Any slow-acting doses will need to be monitored and may need to be altered after a few weeks. Consult your diabetic nurse or GP before changing any dose.

Clear your cupboards, fridge and freezer

Now that you understand what you should be eating and avoiding, set aside some time for a food clear-out. There's nothing more liberating than getting rid of the old to create space for the new, whether clearing out your cupboards or taking a personal inventory. A 'clearing' ritual will signify your decision to commit to a healthier and happier you.

To successfully abstain from all sugar and grains is no easy challenge. It's crucial to clear out your fridge, freezer and cupboards and to replace all the 'junk' with nourishing foods. Don't even attempt to keep sugary or starchy junk food in the house; sometimes no amount of willpower will stop you reaching for whatever foods you are craving.

The excuse of having children or a spouse is not acceptable; it will do them no harm to cut out processed and empty food. Make sure to have a conversation with your family about what you are going to be doing. Explain how important it is that if they want to eat foods that you are looking to exclude, to do it outside the home environment. Make a copy of all the foods that you can have and stick this up in a place that everyone can see.

Get rid of:
- biscuits (sweet and savoury)
- crackers, crisps and pretzels
- baked goods
- chocolates and sweets (please don't use these as 'treats' for your kids)
- bread (even wholewheat and rye)
- pasta and rice
- processed foods
- anything with ingredients you can't identify
- anything with added sugar
- foods labelled 'low-fat' or 'fat-free'
- margarine
- sugar, honey and syrups
- fizzy drinks and any drinks labelled 'sugar-free'.

Enjoy the process of clearing out. You may want to plan a Saturday or Sunday afternoon for the ritual. Remember you're choosing to fill yourself with food that nourishes you. You deserve the best.

Now let's go shopping: stock up on these LCHF basics

It's important to make sure that your kitchen is fully stocked with foods for your LCHF lifestyle. Having these foods available will help whenever a craving comes. Eggs, coconut oil and nut butters will be staples of your diet. Remember that the aim of this lifestyle is to live authentically, so select foods and produce as close to their natural state as possible.

Meat/Fish

Chicken – whole, breast, thighs

Duck

Turkey – all meats and mince

White fish such as halibut, hake, sea bass

Mackerel

Salmon – all varieties, including canned and smoked salmon

Trout

Sardines – canned or fresh

Tuna – canned or fresh

Prawns

Squid

Beef – mince, stewing beef, roasts, steaks

Pork – chops, loin, ribs, roasts

Bacon

Lamb – all meats and mince

Venison and other game

Offal

Ham, Parma ham

Cured meats, salami, pastrami

Vegetables

Artichokes

Asparagus

Aubergines

Avocado

Baby corn

Beansprouts

Broccoli

Brussels sprouts

Cabbage – all varieties

Cauliflower

Celeriac

Celery

Courgettes

Cucumber

Fennel

Green beans

Kale

Leeks

Lettuce – all varieties

Mangetout

Mushrooms

Onions and spring onions

Pak choi

Peppers – green, red, yellow

Rocket

Shallots

Spinach

Tomatoes

Watercress

Dairy/Eggs

Eggs

Milk – whole

Cream

Crème fraîche

Cheese – all hard cheeses, feta and halloumi

Cream cheese

Full-fat Greek or natural yogurt

Sour cream

Unsweetened almond milk

Unsweetened coconut milk

Fats

Almond flour

Coconut flour

Coconut oil

Butter

Almond butter

Cashew butter

Olive oil (use for salads rather than for cooking)

Olives

Ghee

Guacamole

Nuts – almonds, brazils, hazelnuts, macadamias, walnuts

Seeds – chia, linseed (flaxseed), pumpkin, sunflower

Coconut – unsweetened flakes, shredded or desiccated

Dense vegetables

Sweet potato

Carrots

Parsnips

Turnips

Pumpkin

Peas

Sweetcorn

Beetroot

Butternut squash

Fruits

Strawberries

Blackberries

Blueberries

Raspberries

Rhubarb

Lemons

Limes

Herbs/Spices

Allspice

Basil

Bay leaves

Caraway seeds

Cardamom pods

Cayenne pepper

Celery seed

Chillies, chilli powder

Chives

Cinnamon

Coriander – fresh and ground

Cumin

Curry powder

Dill

Dried mixed herbs

Garam masala

Garlic

Ginger

Mustard

Nutmeg

Oregano

Paprika

Parsley

Rosemary

Sage

Sea salt

Black peppercorns

Thyme

Turmeric

Vanilla pods

How to read food labels

Although we want you to get into the habit of cooking most of your meals from scratch, it would be unrealistic to think that you will never consume anything that is out of a packet. If you live a hectic life, we understand that being able to eat on the go is really important.

When reading a food label, make sure that you look at the total carbohydrate content, not just the sugars. Most labels will also list the carbohydrate content per 100g. As a golden rule, never choose anything that has more than 4g per 100g and have no more than a 300g portion of the product.

Typical nutrition information per 100g	
Energy	2673kJ
	645kcal
Fat	54.5g
of which saturates	7.2g
Carbohydrate	9.2g
of which sugars	4.2g
Fibre	6.5g
Protein	26.3g
Salt	1.0g

From a health shop: Almond flour, coconut flour, nut flour, flaxseed meal (ground flaxseeds/linseeds), psyllium husks, chia seeds, cacao powder. Coconut oil and other nut oils. Sugar-free nut butters, for example almond, cashew, macadamia nut, peanut butter, walnut butter.

Dairy: Ghee (some supermarkets sell large tubs, health shops sell smaller quantities).

Other groceries: Mustard, bicarbonate of soda, buttermilk, canned chopped tomatoes, coconut milk and cream, full-fat mayonnaise, olives, Thai curry pastes (green and red), soy sauce, tahini and tomato purée (paste). Vinegars: white wine, cider and balsamic. Meat, chicken or vegetable stock (or make your own).

Legumes (for vegetarians): Soya beans, dry or canned chickpeas, dry or canned beans, lentils, quinoa, frozen soya mince.

Fruit: Fresh fruit, preferably seasonal and locally sourced, is obviously a better choice for dessert or an occasional snack than cakes, pastries or biscuits. However, it is still high in sugar and some people find that it encourages sugar cravings. Keep fruit as an occasional treat and limit yourself to one piece of fruit per day.

Snacks: Biltong, seeds (sunflower, pumpkin, flaxseeds/linseeds, sesame).

Karen

Journaling is one of the greatest tools in my recovery toolkit. I can do it anywhere, at any time. I used to carry a journal around with me and whenever a thought, feeling or idea popped into my head, I'd write it down and so let it out. Now I have a couple of writing apps on my mobile phone, easily accessible and protected with a code.

During emotionally stressful times my head becomes very 'busy'. I find writing down my thoughts and feelings to be a very soothing experience. I allow myself to 'free write'. This is a process I learnt in early recovery: you sit down and just write whatever comes into your mind, no filtering and no judgement. Whenever I do this I feel a great release.

Journal exercise

In Chapters One to Three you may have confronted some issues or a few difficult emotions may have surfaced. Spend a bit of time writing down those feelings. If you're artistically inclined maybe you'd like to draw something instead, or create a simple clay sculpture or piece of art.

Why you should start journaling

We've already asked you to write down answers to questions or to reflect on your feelings in a journal. As part of your recovery programme we'll continue to encourage you to journal frequently, to write down your thoughts and feelings. On a weekly basis we'll also give you exercises and questions to help you reflect on your recovery process.

At the beginning stages of our recovery we found it very useful to list all the food we ate in a daily food diary. We urge you to do this. Find a template at thesugarfreerevolution.com.

As part of the preparation for your journey to recovery you'll need a journal or notebook where you can write down your reflections and answers to the exercises. A simple hardcover exercise book will do – we suggest covering it with inspiring pictures.

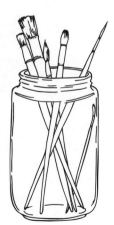

4 Sugar Free recovery model

Throughout this book I will gently guide you on an eight-week journey of empowering yourself in body, mind and spirit. I'll encourage you to challenge your self-limiting and self-defeating thoughts, feelings, beliefs and behaviours. The goal of this programme is to encourage you to be authentic in what you eat, how you behave, what you feel, and how you connect with yourself and others.

Empower body, mind and spirit

My recovery model is based on the premise that we are essentially whole and lack nothing. Through life experiences, interactions with others and traumas, we're led to believe we are lacking and need some external solution to 'fix' us.

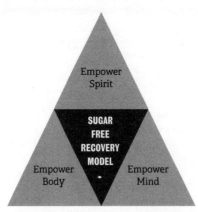

Too many of us live with the underlying belief that 'I'm not good enough', 'I'm not valuable' or 'I'm a failure'. I want you to realise you are good enough, you are valuable and you are a success. You always have been.

My eight-week programme will provide you with tools to empower yourself. You'll pay equal attention to the different parts that make us human beings: body, mind and spirit.

EMPOWER BODY

Meal planning and grocery shopping Learn what, when and how to eat; it sounds simple but you may be amazed at how out of touch many of us have become. Plan your meals in advance, make a shopping list and stick to it, read food labels and stay away from the cake and confectionery aisles. Buy fresh, organic and seasonal veg and fruit – better still, if possible, grow your own. Invest in good-quality meat, butter and dairy – preferably locally sourced.

Mindful eating Turn meal times into a conscious act of love and nourishment. Be present, savour and enjoy.

Ten guiding principles

I developed the Sugar Free manifesto to identify the ten guiding principles by which I live my life.

1 **Quit all sugar.** One day at a time you can do this!

2 **Dream BIG.** Have a vision for yourself and how you want your life to be. Treat life as an adventure and don't settle for mediocrity.

3 **Give your body the foods it deserves.** Think about what you put into your body and understand that you can't out-gym a bad diet.

4 **Move your body.** Perform some form of movement each day and love your body as the unique gift it is. Believe in training smarter, not harder, and know that there is more to life than numbers on the scales.

5 **See health as a lifestyle, not a quick fix.** Choose to be in this for the long haul and embrace the journey of a healthy body, mind and spirit rather than treating it as a destination.

6 **Our thoughts create our reality.** Our internal world shapes our external world. Understand that negative thoughts are just as easily replaceable with positive thoughts and strive to always see the positive in any situation.

7 **Surround yourself with the right people.** The people we spend the most time with play a huge role in our success.

8 **Express gratitude.** Every day. Take time each day to be thankful for the things – no matter how big or small – and people in our lives.

9 **Value experience over stuff.** We know that happiness does not lie within material possessions, but rather in experiences that make us happy.

10 **There is no such thing as failure.** There is only learning. In the same way, the only 'bad' decision is not making a decision in the first place. It is better to act, observe and adjust than to be paralysed into indecision.

Food preparation Good health starts in the kitchen. I will share my favourite recipes and encourage you to experiment and make up your own.

Low-carb eating You have already been introduced to the concept of sugar and carb addiction by neuroscientist Dr Nicole Avena.

Obesity expert and nutritionist Emily Maguire has given you the lowdown on which foods to eat and how to clear your cupboards, fridge and freezer and set yourself up for success. She will also provide you with weekly meal plans that will leave you feeling satisfied and nourished.

Exercise Find something that works for you, that you enjoy, and commit to it. This will involve trial and error. Research the many options available. Challenge yourself and step outside your comfort zone. Exercise is an amazing tool in creating and maintaining health.

EMPOWER MIND

Does your head sometimes feel busy and overcrowded? Let go of the negative clutter and emotional baggage that you are holding on to. Set goals and start working towards them. Remember that there is no quick fix; this programme requires you to commit to yourself and your recovery every moment of the day. Your dedication and action will determine your success. What you put in is what you will get out.

Our emotions, our deepest feelings, serve as guidance systems in our everyday lives. Our emotions help to shape the quality of our experiences and ultimately how successful or unsuccessful we are in achieving our goals.

Throughout this eight-week programme I am going to encourage you to pay attention to your emotions and how you are feeling. You will start the process of acknowledging and understanding your feelings; being able to verbalise them; understanding what triggers certain emotions (and therefore your eating patterns); and learning ways to handle core emotions – fear, shame and guilt – that keep us stuck in addictive patterns.

I do not claim to treat or diagnose any underlying conditions; this book is a self-help tool. Sometimes that may not be enough, and I strongly encourage you to seek professional help or inpatient treatment should you need it. Learning how to ask for help and having your needs met is a very important part of a healthy and happy lifestyle.

EMPOWER SPIRIT

We are human beings not human doings, and during the busyness of our days we often forget the simplicity of being. We pack our schedules to the maximum and leave very little time for nurturing our true essence. It's time to reconnect with your authentic self. Find that inner child and learn how to play. Laugh, love and enjoy life, get back to your natural way of being.

I am going to encourage you to use affirmations that will help you embody the positive ideals you are striving to integrate into your life. At the end of each week I have suggested an affirmation: use it or make up your own. Keep it on hand and say it often.

Enjoy and embrace this process, make yourself the captain of your own life. Keep growing and evolving. The sky is the limit, so spread your wings, take that leap of faith and learn how to fly.

What the eight-week programme looks like

In preparation for your new lifestyle, make sure you've read Chapter Three. Nutritionist Emily Maguire has outlined what you can and can't eat, and explained how the Low Carb Healthy Fat lifestyle can work for vegetarians. It is also important that you clear out your fridge, freezer and cupboards and instead stock them with healthy basics according to the shopping lists provided. The key to success is planning in advance and preparation, so please do not skip this step.

Now you are ready to move on to the eight-week programme:

WEEK 1: FIRST STEPS

I'll help you identify what you need to do to get started on your journey, and how to find help and support. I'll define abstinence, help you understand hunger and explain the ten most important factors for your recovery. At the end of Week One you'll do a check-in and take some simple measurements to use throughout the programme.

WEEK 2: LOW CARB HEALTHY FAT LIFESTYLE

You'll be introduced in more detail to nutritionist Emily Maguire and her journey to the LCHF way of eating. She'll discuss the many benefits of the LCHF lifestyle and how it will work for you. Your family can also be included in the LCHF lifestyle.

WEEK 3: WHO AM I?

I'll encourage you to find a vision for yourself and explore who you really are. You'll get to know your addict personality and learn that it does not define who you are.

WEEK 4: HOW DO I MANAGE MY EMOTIONS?

I'll give you insights into your emotional habits, and tools to help you manage your emotions during your recovery process.

WEEK 5: LOVE MYSELF

Research has shown that all types of addictions (sex, drugs, alcohol, gambling, food) stem from some form of suffering or trauma. The result is that we don't love ourselves. We don't have an accurate sense of ourselves. During Week Five we'll explore ways to boost self-esteem.

WEEK 6: LOVE MY BODY

Exercise is only one part of becoming body-healthy; we also need to love our bodies as they are. This can be difficult to achieve, with the altered images presented in media and advertising. We'll look at how to get more in touch with your body and what it really needs.

WEEK 7: CULTIVATING MINDFULNESS

This eastern spiritual concept has become part of western psychology practices and concepts. We'll examine mindfulness in more detail, and understand why a healthy mind is so important for your recovery and becoming a healthy human being.

WEEK 8: RELAPSE

You aren't perfect. Sometimes you'll have a slip or relapse. But this doesn't mean you are stupid, have no willpower or are never going to 'stay clean'. It just means you had a relapse. During Week Eight we'll explore ways to recover from a relapse, no matter how big.

As I mentioned in Chapter 1 my philosophy is based on five principles:

1
Cut out refined sugar and junk food

2
No refined grains or processed vegetable oils

3
Fat is your friend

4
Great health starts in your kitchen, try to prepare as much as your own food as possible.

5
Empower yourself in body, mind & spirit.

Nutritionist Emily Maguire will provide a meal plan for every week of the programme. You'll also get additional information and journal exercises suited to the topic of the week – based on empowering body, mind and spirit. From Week Two onwards you'll have a peek into someone else's journey into recovery. (A sugar and carb addict wrote each of the anecdotes in this book. Sometimes their names were changed because they prefer to remain anonymous.) There are also tips to deal with difficult situations. At the end of each week, I'll recommend some journal exercises. I also urge you to keep a daily food diary in order to stay accountable and committed to your Sugar Free journey.

At the end of the eight-week programme I'll help you transition your new knowledge and skills into a permanent lifestyle.

To get the most out of this book and to kick-start your journey into recovery, my recommendation is that you work through each week and attempt all exercises and suggestions. And of course you should aim to be Sugar Free from day one. At the beginning of each week, make some time to plan properly: what you're going to eat, when, a schedule for exercise, etc. In Week One we provide some hints and suggestions.

Also, please remember that the success of this programme is determined by the effort that you put in. Your recovery is your responsibility; what you put in is what you will get out.

★

Tips for moving more

Chances are that you have rejected, neglected, ignored and denied your body in too many ways to mention. You may also feel betrayed by your body in one way or another. It's time for this self-destructive body behaviour to stop. Empowering yourself to break free from addiction means empowering yourself in every area of your life, and this includes taking care of your body through exercise.

You may already have an exercise programme that you enjoy – keep it up! But for many people physical exercise is something they last did at school – when they were forced to. Remember that exercise is a positive activity that helps us to bring awareness back to our bodies and away from living in our heads or from our overwhelming emotions. There are some simple things you can do to increase your movement at home, at work or while you are out.

CHAPTER FOUR

What changes could you expect?

Every individual experiences different benefits from this programme. Here is what happened to me.

I started low-carb eating to break the addictive sugar cycle I found myself in. After about a week of sticking to the eating plan I was really surprised by the 'side effects' I experienced:

- Improved and stabilised moods
- Stabilised blood sugar, i.e. no sugar highs followed by crashing lows
- Very few cravings for sugar
- Improved sleep

A couple of weeks down the line I noticed:
- My cellulite had diminished
- Less hunger
- Less water retention
- My weight stabilised, regulated by my own body
- An improvement in my children's eating habits (I was leading by example)
- I felt satiated for prolonged periods after meals
- I was able to distinguish real hunger from emotional hunger
- My skin was clearer, my hair shinier and my nails stronger
- My tastes had changed and I wanted to eat foods that nourished, not diminished me

Remember that these changes take place not only through eating in a LCHF way. They also result from adopting a lifestyle that includes meditation, exercise and paying attention to my body, mind and spirit.

For example:

- Get up from your desk every 20–30 minutes – make yourself some tea or coffee, visit a colleague at their desk.
- Take the stairs wherever you can, or walk up escalators.
- Do a search on the internet for exercises you can do at your desk, and commit to doing these twice a day.
- Park in the furthest corner of the car park.
- Push yourself outside your comfort zone by signing up for a 30-day yoga challenge or entering a body transformation challenge.

Journal excercise

Write down different exercises that you think you will enjoy doing. Think about fun things such as a tango class, hot yoga or even adult ballet classes.

Once you've identified what it is you want to do or explore, write it down and commit to doing it *at least* once a week. Now make the arrangements for doing that one thing. And keep doing that one thing for at least the next eight weeks. At some point you may want to add a second exercise activity. Make sure it's fun and makes you feel fabulous!

Remember if you keep doing the same thing, you'll keep getting the same results. It's time to get healthy, fit and sexy by embracing change and putting yourself out there!

I want to encourage you to find a method of exercise that you not only enjoy but are able to commit to on an ongoing basis. Do not exercise because you feel you have to in order to lose weight or punish yourself. Instead focus on how exercise empowers you – not only your body but your mind, spirit and emotions too. Do it with the knowledge that it makes you healthy and strong.

We are all different: for some people exercise could include walking for 10 minutes every day while others will want to commit

to 45 minutes of yoga three times a week. Exercise can be fun: a dance class with your partner, a paintball session with your friends, getting your children to teach you to skateboard, riding your bike to work, a walk in nature, walking on the beach collecting stones and shells. It is often very helpful to make an exercise date with a friend – it helps you stay committed.

Are you ready to get started?
You probably have questions and concerns to address before you embark on this journey. But first you need to learn a new food equation.

FOOD=FUEL

Food doesn't equal love or caring or happiness or celebration. It's time to start seeing food for what it is: fuel to keep our bodies going. Just as a car needs the right type of fuel to function properly, so do we. Our bodies need different nutrients, vitamins and minerals to function optimally and the foods we eat need to provide these. In Chapter Three, nutritionist Emily Maguire has explained what different types of foods do to our bodies; we've opted for the LCHF or Low Carb Healthy Fat way of eating. Another way of explaining my food philosophy would be to say: Just Eat Real Food. #JERF

Keep it simple, real and authentic in every way.

I'll also help you separate your

Karen

I love the freedom of being outside in nature, so I exercise outdoors as much as possible. It's important to me that my exercise is fun. My favourite activities include running in the forest, exploring the mountains and swimming in the ocean. My family and I often hike at the weekends, making exercise and wellbeing a family affair. For the best stress relief, I take part in some hot and sweaty power yoga. I choose the type of exercise to suit my mood, uplift and empower me.

CHAPTER FOUR

nutritional needs from your emotional needs in order for you to experience a new freedom when it comes to food and eating.

As a child I started identifying specific foods with emotional voids I needed to fill. For example:

Chocolate = safety (my dad used to come home at night with chocolate and his arriving home would make me feel safe).

Toasted cheese sandwiches = comfort (I would try and starve myself at school as I have always imagined my body to be flawed. At about 1 p.m. I just couldn't take the hunger any more and would head on over to the tuck shop for a toasted sarnie, which comforted me).

Pasta = nurturing (when feeling sad or depressed I would cook myself a huge bowl of pasta which would immediately lift my mood).

JOURNAL EXERCISE
What does food mean to you?

Now it's your turn to try and identify the emotional meaning you have given food. Fill in the table below. You'll see that I have added an extra column called action; add an action here that you could use to meet your need that does not involve feeding yourself with food.

Food Example	Food memory What it meant to me	What need or emotion I was trying to meet or soothe?	Action What can I do instead of reaching for that food
Chocolate	Dad's love, safety and security	Safety	Call my dad, ask someone for a hug, journal my feelings, phone a friend

Did you make some startling realisations? Are you shocked at just what a crutch sugar and carbs are to you?

If you're paging through the rest of the book now and thinking 'I really can't do this', or 'I don't have the time' or 'There's too much to do and to think about', please don't give up. This is your addictive personality talking because it's feeling over-whelmed – the emotion is too big. The easy thing is to give up. Your addictive personality doesn't like change and you're challenging it.

I suggest you start small: stick to the meal plans for eight weeks and write your daily food diary. You'll gain so much insight into your own eating patterns if you also work through Week One's pointers – there's helpful advice about dealing with your sugar and carb addiction.

Once you're comfortable with your routine of food and eating, go through the eight-week programme again. This time, read the information and attempt the different exercises. Use this book as a resource to help you in your journey of recovery. It doesn't matter how long it takes – what's important is that you take the first steps and keep on the path.

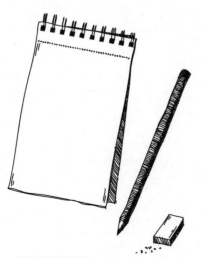

Some things that may still be bothering you

1
If this is not a diet, what should I be doing? You're right – I'm not advocating a diet, I'm advocating a lifestyle change based on authenticity in the way you eat, think, feel and behave. My philosophy can be broken into five simple steps: cut out refined sugar and junk food; no refined grains or processed vegetable oils; fat is your friend; great health starts in your kitchen; try and prepare as much of your own food as possible and lastly, make the time to empower yourself in body, mind & spirit.

My eight-week plan will help you do just that.

2
What do you mean by no sugar? That's what I mean. No added sugar or sweeteners to your tea or coffee. No food containing added sugar such as processed food and baked goods, muffins or cakes. No sweets. No fizzy drinks or fruit juice. No fast food. Keep it real and simple, as close to its natural state as possible, so if you must give in to your chocolate cravings, for example, opt for extra dark, with a cocoa content of at least 70%; and if you fancy an alcoholic drink, consume in extreme moderation, and refer to our list on p26 so you can make an informed choice.

CHAPTER FOUR

3

And you want me to do this from day one? Absolutely! You may not believe that you can do this (yet) but I absolutely do. I know it's hard, I really do. Your heart probably sped up and your mind was flooded with 'but I can't do that' protests. That's just your addictive personality putting barriers in your way, because it is something you can do. Did you know all successful diets (those that help people lose weight) eliminate sugar?

4

I'm not sure I can do that. Go back and reread your health and diet history. I bet you've given up sugar in the past. That means you can do it again. There must be a compelling reason why you bought this book, and decided you were ready for a lifestyle change. Remember that you are not alone! I am with you every step of the way. If you can find a friend or group to work through this book with then even better; there is definitely strength in numbers and you will keep each other motivated along the way.

5

Well, maybe I can. Replace your fruit juice with fruit, put cream in your tea and coffee instead of milk and sugar, and cook with coconut oil, butter and cream. Does that make it a little easier?

6

OK, I think I'm ready to do this. Remember that throughout this programme I'll encourage you to take it one day, one meal at a time. 'Just for today' will become your mantra.

7

Can I eat snacks? Only if you are hungry. Emily's weekly meal plans include a daily snack option.

8

I usually eat snacks while I'm working at my desk. I want you to make a meal out of your food, to eat without distraction. Sit at a table, not in front of the television. This includes your snacks. Take five or ten minutes away from your computer. You can sit at your desk, but eat your snack slowly and enjoy every bite.

9

If this isn't about the scales, how will I know if I'm progressing? To measure your progress you'll be looking at three key areas: your weight, some basic measurements (including your waist circumference) and your overall mood and energy levels. In the 'First steps' chapter of the eight-week programme, I'll take you through these step by step.

10

I'm not sure I can do this for eight weeks. This is not only about the next eight weeks, this is the rest of your life. But I understand – eight weeks seems a very long time. As a first step, why not take a 21-day challenge or join my supportive online forum to keep you motivated and inspired?

11

What do you mean by a 21-day challenge? I challenge you to follow our recommendations and suggestions for 21 days. That's all. I'm quite confident that after sticking to the programme for 21 days you will want to continue for another 21 days. You will feel refreshed, revitalised and renewed.

12

So the 21-day challenge means I have to do three things: Cut sugar and carbohydrates from my diet, move more, and take time to nourish my mind and spirit? Yes. And at the end of the challenge I'd like you to share your story with me on thesugarfreerevolution.com.

13

I already have a vigorous exercise programme. That's great news. Please continue with what works for you. If you notice any changes in your energy levels please consult a healthcare professional.

14

So are you saying I can't eat the foods identified in the journal exercise above? Yes. You have to practise abstinence from the foods you most often use to quell distressing emotions. The food you turn to when you want comfort or

that you use to celebrate. The food you easily overeat. And yes, I'm saying that for the duration of this programme you can't eat it.

15

Will I experience any withdrawal symptoms? You may experience slight physical discomfort like a headache, or cravings for sugar and carbohydrates. But you should notice an improved physical wellbeing after a few days: less bloating and a clearer head, increased energy and improved mood. Need more motivation?

16

What do you mean by no carbohydrates? No grains. No wheat. No pasta. No rice. No sushi (except sashimi, and hold the pickled ginger as it's laden with sugar). No potatoes (except sweet potatoes). No bread.

17

I'm not sure I can do that. What if we show you some delicious alternatives to try – some vegetable options to replace rice and spaghetti? Instead of bread, try wrapping sandwich fillings in lettuce leaves, or using large mushrooms to create a burger 'roll', for instance. There are plenty of great recipes on my blog thesugarfreerevolution.com; you won't get bored. And you can still enjoy sweet potatoes in moderation – a great alternative if you enjoy hot chips.

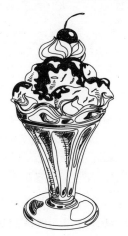

18

No ice cream? No conventional ice cream. But there are some great sugar free recipes online.

19

What if I slip up and give in to temptation? You are human and genetically programmed to over-indulge in sweet things. And you have identified yourself as an addict. I'm not saying a relapse is inevitable but it is possible. I've had to learn to take it one day and one meal at a time. If you do slip up that doesn't mean your next meal has to be a complete disaster. One mistake is just that: one mistake. In Week Eight I address relapses in more detail. You can jump to that section and read it now if that's a concern.

20

I'm excited about starting and I want to learn more. I am so excited that you have chosen to commit yourself and your health. Welcome to the rest of your life. I am with you every step of the way and will provide you with loads of resources in this book that will help you on your journey.

21

So this lifestyle change is just about giving up sugar and carbs, right? Giving up sugar and carbs is only part of learning the new food equation: food equals fuel. I'll also give you tools to help you deal with your emotions, cravings and addictive behaviour. That includes exercise.

22

I've tried similar things before. What will be different this time? Remember two things: sugar is addictive. Addiction is a disease that is chronic and progressive unless recovery is sought. As scary as this may sound there is a solution and recovery is possible!

23

What do I still need to do to be ready? It sounds as if you're ready right now to start the eight-week programme. In the next chapter, I'll help you to take the first steps to become Sugar Free and create your own health revolution!

5 First steps – laying a firm foundation

Getting started with a new habit can be a daunting task. Research has shown it can take anything from a week to a year to establish a habit – its success depends on the pattern you're trying to create and your personal history. In recovery from addiction, prolonged abstinence can be determined by the strength of the foundation you lay. Just as a house needs a solid foundation on which to be built, so do we. This week is all about identifying what's needed to create that foundation and then doing it.

Only you can choose to set yourself up for success.

Ten important factors for your recovery

1 PLANNING AND PREPARATION
Planning and preparation are key to success. Plan your meals in advance; if possible set aside some time on a Sunday to prepare as many meals as possible in advance. Also remember to stock your fridge and freezer. Schedule time for your exercise and stick to it no matter what. Get into a routine and adhere to it. This is the most effective tool for your recovery. Take 30 minutes at the weekend and plan the week ahead.

● What will you be eating, when and where?
● Do you have that food in your cupboard or fridge or do you need to go shopping?
● Are there any meals that you can prepare in advance to be frozen or stored?
● If you'll be out during a meal-time can you easily order LCHF dishes? Or should you take snacks?
● Will you exercise in the morning or evening? How many times will you be exercising?
● Are you going to exercise on your own, in a class or with a friend?
● Have you planned a nurturing activity for yourself? A long hot bath, some quiet time, or making a gratitude list?
● Have you scheduled a fun activity? A treat that does not involve food.

If you have a plan when you're trying to lose weight and get fit, you're more likely to stick to a healthy-eating pattern and lifestyle. We've created an eating plan for each of the eight weeks of the programme: use these as the foundation for your LCHF way of life.

2 SAY NO TO SUGAR
And keep a look out for hidden sugar in the most unexpected places. I encourage you to stay away from artificial sweeteners such as aspartame, Splenda and Canderel, etc. and 'natural' sweeteners such as stevia, xylitol and agave. Avoid diet drinks too.

Karen

When I started living the low-carb lifestyle I cut out all refined sugar. I still included fruit though – fruits high in sugar such as mango, grapes and watermelon, which left me craving more of not only those fruits but any sugar. I now limit my fruit intake and don't include it daily. Finding what works for you is a process of trial and error. Increasing my fat intake also really helped my sugar cravings. Now when I crave sugar I often have a spoonful of coconut oil; it takes away the physical craving instantly.

3 FIND A FRIEND, GROUP OR COMMUNITY TO WORK THROUGH THIS BOOK WITH
There is great power in a group. You'll boost your recovery by having other people witness your story, by sharing tools and recipes, and by helping others with their recovery. This can be my online programme, an Overeaters Anonymous group that meets weekly, or a group that you have managed to get together to work through this book.

Identifying with others helps us recognise our common problems, and witnessing other recoveries makes it clear that rehabilitation

from sugar and carb addiction is possible. Remember: you are not alone.

Some of us need more than a recovery community or group of friends for support. Don't be afraid to seek professional help. If you're struggling with what to eat, see a nutritionist or registered dietitian sympathetic to the LCHF way of eating. Please make sure that the person you are asking for help is university degree-qualified and an expert in their field. Working with a psychologist or counsellor on a one-on-one basis can also provide a greater understanding of you, your behaviours and relationships. Always consult a medical practitioner for any medical advice.

4 EDUCATE YOURSELF
Find ways to help yourself connect with your new lifestyle. There's a lot of information about low-carb high-fat lifestyles on the internet. If you enjoy social media then join me on Facebook, Twitter and Instagram sharing your recipes, meals, successes and struggles. You'll soon find other websites and newsletters. Throughout this book I'll suggest resources helpful to your recovery.

5 REMEMBER THIS IS AN EMPOWERED LIFESTYLE CHANGE
This is not a diet. This is a lifestyle. And while it may be for the rest of your life, take it one day and one meal at a time. You want progress, not perfection.

6 ONE SLIP DOESN'T MAKE YOU A BAD PERSON

Or a person who is out of control. Or someone who can never stick to things. Or useless. Or crazy. You just made a mistake. Use it as an opportunity to learn what to do differently in the future.

7 TAKE TIME FOR YOURSELF EVERY DAY

One way to do this is by writing in a journal. Even if it's only 10 minutes a day. I'll provide useful journal exercises throughout the book. One of the greatest tools in my recovery is a gratitude journal and I make sure I list ten things I am grateful for at least once a day. What we focus on grows, so focus on gratitude and draw more positivity into your life.

8 LEARN TO MEDITATE

Meditation helps you get closer to your own thoughts. I'll explore meditation and mindfulness in Week Seven (Cultivating mindfulness). Did you know meditation isn't only sitting in one place and closing your eyes? Yoga, going for a walk in nature or walking the dog are all forms of meditation. You can make a meditative practice out of washing the dishes or the car. Meditation is simply a space where you pay attention to the moment and observe your own thoughts.

9 UNDERSTAND YOUR TRIGGERS

Our emotions, people and situations can trigger us to turn to food to soothe ourselves. What triggers one person may not have the same effect on somebody else. It's important to identify your triggers as well as comfort or binge foods and abstain from them completely. Have a plan as to how you'll deal with them. I'll discuss this in more detail later in this chapter. Also understand that trigger foods will change over time, so it's important to be vigilant and honest with yourself regarding your addictive behaviour.

10 LOVE YOURSELF

Start right now. You're a beautiful, capable and worthwhile person just as you are. Self-love is the greatest gift you can give yourself and others. Embrace your imperfections and idiosyncrasies; they are what make you unique and beautiful.

Affirmations

Many people have difficulty in accepting themselves as worthwhile and lovable. Affirmations are a way of 're-programming' your brain to help you think and act in a more positive way. By holding yourself in high esteem you give others the permission to do the same. Find an affirmation that resonates with you and repeat it as often as possible.

Karen

One of the most useful things for my recovery was identifying my triggers and finding solutions for them (not 'feeding' them with sugar). I know I need to HALT when I'm feeling Hungry, Angry, Lonely and/or Tired.

When I'm feeling hungry I ask myself: Am I physically hungry right now or is my hunger of an emotional origin? Do I need food or a hug, compassion, kindness or love? I feed the need and not the feeling. Anger is a big trigger for me. Whether angry with others or myself I tend to punish myself by using food to self-medicate. I now take time out by going to sit somewhere quietly and breathing, or going for a walk or run. Loneliness makes me feel very sorry for myself, and once again run to the fridge or corner shop for sweet comfort. So now I meet friends, go to a movie or get outside. Feeling tired is my worst form of self-punishment. Even though it's not always avoidable, planning ahead ensures that I accommodate my need for rest and sleep.

Some examples of affirmations:

- I am good enough as I am.
- I am beautiful inside and out.
- Today I love and accept myself exactly as I am.
- I have everything I need within me, I don't need to reach for food.
- I deserve love and happiness.

I will be providing you with an affirmation at the end of every week. Use mine or make up your own. Affirm the positive in yourself and watch it grow. You are worth it.

Getting help and support
You can't do this on your own. There are support groups such as Overeaters Anonymous and Sugar Addicts Anonymous to join, but remember you already have your own personal support group set up. 'I have?' is probably the question you're pondering. Of course you do – your family and friends already care about you. Although they may not understand what it means to be a sugar and carb addict, they certainly understand you. It's up to you to educate them about your journey and your goal to become free of sugar and carbs.

Step one
Make a list of all the people you need support from:

- Husband, wife, lover or life partner
- Children
- Parents
- Friends
- Work colleagues
- Any friend or team that you walk, run or play sport with
- Book club

Step two
Read through the letter I've provided on the next page. Amend and add to it. Make it your own. You may want to write variations for certain people.

Step three
Fax, email, text, tweet, Facebook, blog or handwrite your letter. There are endless ways in which you can communicate your intention and ask for support and help. You may just inspire someone else to join your journey.

Learning to say no to sugar
The thought of cutting all sugar and processed carbohydrates out of your life may seem a daunting task. Remember I'm only asking you to commit one day at a time. Think of it even more simply – one moment at a time. Not only do you need to retrain your taste buds, but also the way you think about yourself and value your worth. Every day you need to consciously commit to your recovery. You hold the power to say no until the point that you put sugar into your mouth.

Always keep my equation FOOD = FUEL at the forefront of your mind. If you are craving sugar and carbs and have no biological reason for needing fuel then ask yourself what is really going on. Identify the need and fill it appropriately.

Surrounding yourself with people, places and things that are supportive and conducive to your sugar and carbohydrate abstinence is probably the most important part of this journey.

Creating a home environment that is Sugar Free is simple enough. In Chapter Three we helped you to clean out your cupboards, fridge and freezer. When you go shopping, keep it simple. Start at the veggie section, proceed to meat and dairy and then to the checkout. There's no need to venture anywhere near the bread, pasta or sweet aisles. When standing in queues surrounded by infinite sweet temptations, keep yourself occupied by skimming a magazine or checking your emails until it's your turn to pay. Another option is to order your food online and have it delivered: this saves time and keeps you away from temptation. In Week Two I will give you tips on helping your kids become Sugar Free.

The most challenging situations usually present themselves when you're with people who don't know you're abstaining from sugar and carbohydrates. Say, for instance, you're invited to someone's house

Dear

Over the next eight weeks I'm embarking on a personal journey to cut out sugar and carbohydrates in my diet. I want to make a lifestyle change for my health.

When I eat sugar or carbohydrates I start feeling out of control. I sometimes become moody and upset. I am often riddled with shame and guilt. I also start craving more and more of them. The negative consequences from eating sugar and carbs far outweigh the positive and therefore I want to abstain in the future.

Personal success doesn't come without support. In other words, I need your help. If you invite me over for supper/lunch/breakfast please don't be offended if:

- I contact you to find out what's on the menu. This is me taking care of myself and ensuring that I have access to food I want to eat.
- I refuse dessert – I know you made it especially for me because I love desserts, but to use an old cliché, they don't love me. What about asking me to bring dessert? I know some great healthy alternatives.
- I don't eat your delicious pasta dish and enjoy the salad instead.
- I don't eat the bread.

Also, please don't buy me chocolates or cake as a way of saying thank you. If I say no to birthday cake it's not because I don't like you – I'm just taking care of myself. If I get moody or irritated it's not you – I'm probably experiencing withdrawal symptoms. If you see me reaching for chocolate or a piece of cake, please stop me. This is my sugar and carb addict wanting a fix. Ask me: 'What are you feeling right now?' or 'What do you really want?' I may be grumpy at the time but I'll thank you later. I know you love having treats (chocolates, cake or biscuits) in the house or office. But I won't be able to control myself and will want to eat them. Please will you lock them in a cupboard and keep the key.

With your support and encouragement I know I will be able to make these changes in my life. My goal is to be healthy and to live a happy and abundant life.

I am learning to fight for myself; I want the very best life has to offer. Thank you for your support, it means the world to me.

---

*
A note on deprivation

Feeling deprived could possibly be the greatest obstacle in your recovery from sugar and carb addiction. Feeling deprived could lead to rebellion, resentment and ultimately lapsing and not returning to the Sugar Free programme.

Instead of seeing your recovery as a forced deprivation from sugar and carbs, look at it as a way of empowering your health. Instead of saying: 'I am not allowed sugar' say 'I am choosing my health and wellbeing by filling myself with nourishing foods'. Change your mindset, change your life – it really can be as simple as that.

JOURNAL EXERCISE

Take a few moments to write down a few difficult
scenarios you may be confronted with and some ways
you could deal with them. In the abstinence and hunger
sections later in this chapter, we'll help you identify
other coping mechanisms.

LIFE SCENARIO	WHAT WILL I SAY?
Offered cake, biscuits or chocolate at the office	No thank you, I don't eat sugar.
Pressurised by a friend to have 'just one' because 'What harm can it do?'	Thank you, but no thank you.

Karen

When I first stopped eating sugar I used the phrase 'No
thank you, I don't eat sugar' when refusing anything with
sugar in it – chocolate, cake, biscuits, etc. It was easy.
Most people just said 'Oh' and moved on to offer the food
to somebody else.

As with other chemical and behavioural addictions the
most important thing is to not take that first hit of your
drug. When you do experience a craving, try to delay that
urge by a couple of minutes. Every moment you delay
that first bite will be a victory in itself. Ask for help by
phoning a friend, logging on to a supportive online group
or moving away from the temptation. In the beginning
it will be tough, but one day you'll find you've changed
those taste buds and a once-powerful substance holds
very little appeal (yes, it does happen).

for dinner, have a food-related work function or have to meet somebody for lunch in a restaurant. Peer pressure can be one of the greatest challenges, especially if people aren't aware that you're trying to change your lifestyle.

You have two choices: either share your story and ask for support, or keep it to yourself and put up very firm boundaries. The best advice we can give you is to say 'No' when you're offered sugar or carbohydrates. No is a complete sentence. You don't have to explain yourself to anyone. Remember you're putting your recovery first. What you think about yourself is far more important than what others think.

Why abstinence is so important

One is too many and a thousand never enough. As addicts, once we start eating sugar we can't stop. We use sugar and carbs to numb ourselves, to soothe our feelings. We use them to avoid confronting what is upsetting us, or making us angry or sad. Sugar and carbs become a substitute for feeling, for growing as a human being. Yes, we could tell ourselves we're only going to have one slice of bread or one small chocolate – but before we know it the whole loaf is gone or the box of chocolates is finished.

Why? We believe the commitments or promises we make to ourselves about sugar and carbs. We buy into the stories we spin about our addiction:

'I'm only going to have one.'

'I'm only going to have this once.'

'I won't have any tomorrow.'

'I'll start eating properly on Monday.'

'It won't hurt to have one now.'

But it's very difficult to admit we don't have the ability to control our behaviour around sugar and carbs, despite the overwhelming evidence that tells us differently. We are not in control. Denial is just a self-defence mechanism, a means of protecting ourselves from the painful truth of addiction. A way to break that denial is to practise abstinence. By abstinence I mean avoiding foods, behaviours, thoughts and situations that could lead to overeating and bingeing on sugar and carbs.

Abstinence is a core part of your recovery. Recovery is the complete opposite of addiction: we don't run away from our problems, we face them. We don't ignore the voice of pain inside us, we listen to it. Recovery is about restoring your true self.

But abstinence from what? Unlike other addictions, with any food addiction you can't stop eating food; food nourishes the body physically.

Do you remember that food equation?

FOOD=FUEL

We need fuel for our bodies and minds to function.

Only you can decide which foods and behaviours you need to abstain from to ensure your recovery. Think about the situations and foods that lead to overeating. Or the behaviours and foods that lead to overindulging in sugar and carbs, behaviours seductive enough to interfere with your recovery.

Start by returning to the personal weight history you outlined in Chapter One. Read through it and think about your eating patterns and history.

What are your food triggers?
Anybody addicted to sugar or carbohydrates has an underlying belief that these foods will make them feel better.

Do these statements sound familiar?

'I've had a hard day at the office so I'll just stop off at the corner shop and buy some chocolate.'

'My boss just yelled at me so I'm going to have an extra slice of that birthday cake.'

'I deserve that extra helping of dessert – I worked hard in the garden.'

Karen

My biggest trigger is feeling rejected. My first modelling job was at the age of five, and after going to what feels like thousands of castings, rejection has played a big role in my life. When I have a disagreement with a loved one or work colleague I take it personally and all my old feelings of low self-worth start to resurface. In that moment all I want is a little comfort – where better to turn than a chocolate or cola? In recovery I've had to learn how to say no and put up very firm boundaries. I've had to learn to love and accept myself as I am (feeling, thinking and being) in that moment. That has truly been my greatest gift.

Triggers, abstinence and recovery

Spend some time writing down answers to the following questions:

1 When do you eat?

2 Where do you eat?

3 Why do you eat?

4 Who are your eating partners (certain people may make it harder to say no to second helpings or dessert)?

5 What are your favourite restaurants?

6 Which places trigger your eating compulsion (it could be a supermarket)?

7 Do your activities have an effect (some people are tempted to binge after a workout session because they've 'worked so hard' and 'deserve it')?

8 Any other trigger situations (such as having a fight with a family member)?

9 Do you have favourite places in the house where you binge or overindulge (in bed or tucked up on your sofa)?

10 Are there particular emotions (fear, shame and guilt) that lead you to reach for your favourite food?

11 Are there foods you can't stop eating once you start? Or foods that trigger you to eat other sugar- and carb-laden items?

12 Are there particular foods you choose to binge on?

13 Have you experienced negative consequences as a result of your sugar and carb addiction? How has it affected your health? Relationships with others as well as yourself?

14 Do you consume sugar and carbs in a way that is shameful and embarrassing? Do you hide your consumption from others?

Now take this list and decide which situations, behaviours and foods you need to abstain from to aid your recovery. Use the following diagram to chart them:

In the inner circle, put all those foods, behaviours and situations that you wish to abstain from.

In the middle circle, put all those foods, behaviours and situations that would lead you to indulge in sugar and carbs.

In the outer circle, put all those behaviours you consider to be healthy and contributing towards your recovery.

Karen

My cravings for sugar are strongest when I'm feeling emotionally 'down'. During these times when I'm feeling angry, lonely or sad, I want to soothe myself with a huge bowl of pasta and cola, followed by a slab of chocolate and some sweets. Instead of indulging in these behaviours I'll see what I can do to soothe myself that is not related to food. I practise SOS, which stands for Stop, Observe and Steer. I stop and breathe, observe what's going on and find the best possible solution to 'feed' myself emotionally while steering away. Often this includes surrounding myself in nature, going for a walk, writing in my journal or phoning a recovery friend. I try to have at least three options for every trigger I've identified.

I also find grocery shopping with my kids very stressful, but this is often avoidable if I plan my week in advance. Another solution is shopping online via my local organic market's website. The goods are delivered straight to my door.

I abstain from the following:

1 Sugar

2 Eating to soothe, reward or punish myself

3 Junk food in any form

4 Processed food

5 Most products associated with a TV advertisement

6 Anything containing ingredients I cannot pronounce, so most colourings and additives

7 Artificial sweeteners, or any person or thing that seems artificial

8 Fruit, most of the time

To help you get started, here are my circles.

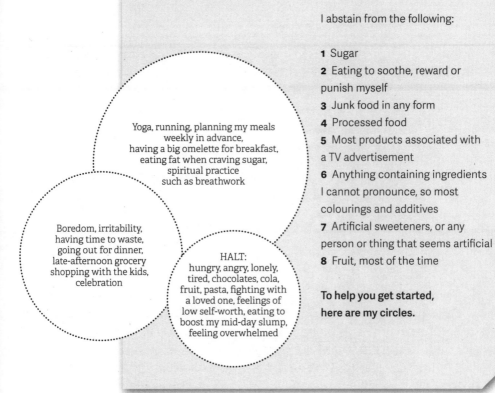

Yoga, running, planning my meals weekly in advance, having a big omelette for breakfast, eating fat when craving sugar, spiritual practice such as breathwork

Boredom, irritability, having time to waste, going out for dinner, late-afternoon grocery shopping with the kids, celebration

HALT: hungry, angry, lonely, tired, chocolates, cola, fruit, pasta, fighting with a loved one, feelings of low self-worth, eating to boost my mid-day slump, feeling overwhelmed

How will you define your abstinence?

Take a few moments to reflect on your weight history and the answers to the abstinence questions on p55. Write a list of all the activities and foods from which you will be abstaining. You may want to date and sign this list. It's a good idea to share it with someone who'll support you in your recovery. When you think about abstinence, don't think about it as saying no to certain behaviours, situations or food. Rather think about it as saying YES to abstinence and to your recovery.

Turning a feeling of deprivation into an empowered step is a powerful tool in changing your mindset from being addiction-seeking to being recovery-focused. When I am feeling deprived and angry that I am not allowed loose in the chocolate aisle, I write down my choice as follows:

Today I CHOOSE to fill my body with healthy and nourishing foods and thoughts. I deserve the very best life has to offer. This is my choice.

Are you really hungry?

We eat to cover our emotions, and to deal with pain and frustrations. In doing this we've lost touch with our bodies and two very important body signals:

1 Am I hungry?
2 Am I full?

Many of us don't know the answers to those questions. So I'm suggesting you create some boundaries for yourself around your eating:

1
Always place your food on a plate or in a bowl. Or if you're preparing food in advance, make sure your portion is contained in, for example, a ziplock snack bag.

2
Always sit and eat your food in a designated eating place (at home or work) away from distractions.

3
Eat breakfast, lunch and supper (under-eating can be a trigger for overeating).

4

Plan for your two snacks (these aren't compulsory).

5

Get into a routine of specific times of day when you eat, and plan your meals for three to four hours apart.

6

Plan your week in advance.

7

Measure your fats. Weigh your proteins. Weigh your heavy vegetables. Measure your fruit.

8

Write down what you've eaten on a daily basis. You can also use an app on your phone to record this information.

Sometimes we want second helpings directly after we've eaten, or we get hungry in between meals. How do you know if your body is still hungry or whether it is only your emotions wanting to be fed?

The next time you're hungry, use this checklist to help you identify true hunger:

1

When did I last eat? Was it a few hours ago? So is it time for my next meal or snack?

2

If the answer is 'No' have a glass of water and wait 20 minutes. Then ask, 'Am I still hungry?'

3

Ask, 'If I ate something now would this satisfy me?'

If you answered 'Yes' to any of these questions then you're probably physically hungry so it's a good idea to eat.

4

Now ask yourself, 'How physically hungry am I?' and look at these responses:

a Not hungry
b Slightly empty
c Empty
d Hungry
e Very hungry
f Very, very hungry
g Starving and irritable
h Weak and faint

You should aim to eat when you feel empty (for a snack) or hungry to very hungry (for a meal). If you're eating when you aren't hungry then you're probably practising emotional eating. If you keep your hunger at bay until you're overly hungry or starving, this could trigger overeating or reaching for foods that feed your sugar and carb addiction.

If you answered 'No' to any of questions 1–3 above then you're emotionally eating to feel better about yourself or the situation you're in.

Answer these questions to help you identify what it is you really need instead of food:

5
What am I feeling right now?
- Bored
- Anxious
- Sad
- Lonely
- Tired
- Overwhelmed
- Stressed
- Angry

6
What can I do right now to manage my feelings?

JOURNAL EXERCISE
What can you do instead of eating?

Write a list of all the things you could be doing instead of eating. Here are suggestions to consider:

- Call someone who always makes you feel better.
- Play with your dog or cat.
- Look at a favourite photo or cherished memento.
- Interact with your children.
- Dance to your favourite song.
- Squeeze a stress ball.
- Take a brisk walk.
- Treat yourself to a hot cup of tea.
- Take a bath.
- Light some scented candles.
- Wrap yourself in a cosy blanket.
- Read a good book.
- Watch a comedy show.
- Explore the outdoors.
- Turn to an activity you enjoy (woodworking, playing the guitar, scrapbooking, etc.).
- Meditate or pray.
- Look up a daily reading from a spiritual book.

Revisit the journal exercise in Chapter Four on what your food means to you and add anything you may have missed or have just become aware of.

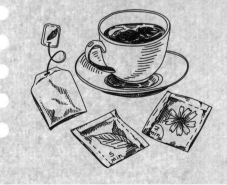

Karen

One of my fondest childhood memories is of my dad going to the shop in the evenings to buy us a treat. He always bought me a Cadbury's Flake chocolate and I'd delight in every bite. That gesture of specially going to the shop and buying something sweet made me feel loved and supported. No surprise then that when I'm feeling unloved or unsupported, I want to rush to the shop to buy chocolate. What I should do instead is to identify why I'm feeling unloved and unsupported, and then figure out how to have those needs met. Depending on the support I need, I can ask somebody for a hug, have a long bath, go for a walk, sit quietly and breathe, or write about my feelings.

Can you tell the difference between emotional and physical hunger?

EMOTIONAL HUNGER	PHYSICAL HUNGER
Starts suddenly.	Comes on gradually.
Is often a craving – feels like it needs to be satisfied immediately.	The feeling can often wait.
Usually craves those comfort foods you put in the middle of your abstinence circles.	When you're physically hungry you're open to options – lots of things look tasty and sound satisfying.
Is never satisfied, even when your stomach is full.	It stops when you are full.
When you eat to satisfy an emotion it triggers feelings of guilt, regret, powerlessness and shame.	Eating to satisfy physical hunger doesn't make you feel bad about yourself.
Can lead to mindless eating.	This eating fuels your body.
This craving can feel like you can't get it out of your head – you become fixated on specific foods, tastes and textures.	It's located in your body – a growling or a pang in your stomach.

Week One check-in

As you begin your journey it's a good idea to take a few basic measurements and track them over time. Our suggestion is to measure now and at the end of eight weeks (we'll remind you).

If you are still looking to lose weight or body fat, then maintaining a carbohydrate level of 50g or less is advisable. (Once you have achieved your weight-loss goal and maintained it for a minimum of one month you might look at making adjustments.) This level of carbohydrate intake would also be advisable for diabetics and individuals who are insulin resistant or have problems with blood sugar levels. In order to determine this, we would recommend that you have your blood sugar measured regularly throughout the programme. If your levels remain high (or low), then staying at 50g would probably be best for you. You can use a blood glucose checker available from high-street pharmacies or online, or visit your GP/practice nurse. If you are diabetic and/or are on medication, then do not make any changes to your diet or treatment without first seeking medical advice.

If you're doing the 21-day challenge mentioned in Chapter Four, we'll remind you to measure at 21 days. Of course, anyone is welcome to do so at 21 days anyway.

MEASUREMENT	BEGINNING WEEK ONE	21 DAYS	END OF WEEK EIGHT
Weigh yourself. At the gym, at the doctor or at home.			
Take your waist measurement. This is the narrowest point on your torso.			
Take your hip measurement. Feel for your hipbones and measure across the widest part.			
(If female) Take your bust measurement. Take two measurements: under your bust and across your breasts.			
What are your overall energy levels? Rate out of 10 (0 is no energy and 10 is on top of the world).			
What is your mood generally? Mostly irritable and annoyed? Do you look forward to the day or feel grumpy when you wake up? Reflect on this in your journal.			

WEEKLY JOURNAL EXERCISE

Take a few minutes to reflect on your week and this stage of your journey:

1. What were your greatest successes this week?
2. How will you build on your successes?
3. Did you stick to your meal plan?
4. Did you maintain abstinence from sugar and carbs?
5. If not, what triggered you to relapse or slip?
   What have you learnt from this experience?
6. What exercise did you do this week?
7. Are you unhappy about anything that happened this week?
8. Have you been affirming yourself?
9. What will you do differently next week to support
   your journey in recovery positively?
10. Make a list of ten things you are grateful for.

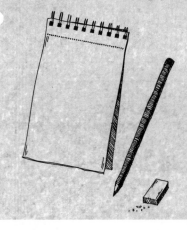

Affirmation

I deserve the very best life has to offer.

USEFUL RESOURCES

Addictive Thinking: Understanding Self-Deception (second edition) by Abraham J. Twerski (Hazelden, 1997). How self-deceptive thought can undermine self-esteem and threaten the sobriety of a recovering addict.

The Addictive Personality: Understanding the Addictive Process and Compulsive Behaviour by Craig Nakken (Hazelden, 1996). Bringing new insights to understandings of how somebody becomes an addict, Nakken uncovers the common denominator of all addictions.

				DAY 1
Breakfast	**Lunch**	**Dinner**	**Snacks**	**Drinks**
3 tbsp natural whole-milk (or Greek) yogurt mixed with 1 tbsp double cream (optional), 1 tbsp coconut flakes, 30g mixed nuts and 50g berries	Tuna Niçoise Salad (see recipe)	Coconut Chicken (see recipe) with mango, chilli salsa, served with a large green salad	**Consume up to 2 snacks per day and only when hungry** 10 olives Up to 30g hard cheese 10 Parmesan Crisps with 1 tbsp homemade Guacamole or homemade salsa ½ an avocado topped with balsamic vinegar 50g nuts (not peanuts) 1 Fat Bomb	6–8 glasses of water Tea and coffee (herbal or decaf if you prefer) In coffee and tea, try sticking with double cream or unsweetened almond or coconut milk

				DAY 2
Egg, salmon and avocado platter: 3 eggs (cooked any way you like), 50g salmon (any kind), ½ an avocado and 6 cherry tomatoes	Chicken Tikka Strips (see recipe) served on a large bed of spinach, 50g cucumber and 8 cherry tomatoes with 1 tbsp crème fraîche on top	1 small steak (about 100g) served with a creamy mushroom sauce served with one handful of green beans cooked in 2 tsp butter	**Consume up to 2 snacks per day and only when hungry** 10 olives Up to 30g hard cheese 10 Parmesan Crisps with 1 tbsp homemade Guacamole or homemade salsa ½ an avocado topped with balsamic vinegar 50g nuts (not peanuts) 1 Fat Bomb	6–8 glasses of water Tea and coffee (herbal or decaf if you prefer) In coffee and tea, try sticking with double cream or unsweetened almond or coconut milk

				DAY 3
Sugar-free Granola (see recipe) (50g) with either unsweetened almond milk or 3 tbsp of Greek yogurt with 50g berries	Up to 5 salmon wraps: smoked salmon strips (up to 75g) spread with 2 tsp full-fat cream cheese and cucumber slices, rolled up	Chicken Stuffed with Ham and Cheese (see recipe) served with roasted Mediterranean vegetables (aubergine, courgettes, peppers, red onion and tomatoes)	**Consume up to 2 snacks per day and only when hungry** 10 olives Up to 30g hard cheese 10 Parmesan Crisps with 1 tbsp homemade Guacamole or homemade salsa ½ an avocado topped with balsamic vinegar 50g nuts (not peanuts) 1 Fat Bomb	6–8 glasses of water Tea and coffee (herbal or decaf if you prefer) In coffee and tea, try sticking with double cream or unsweetened almond or coconut milk

Breakfast	Lunch	Dinner	Snacks	Drinks
3 rashers of bacon with 50g cream cheese and 50g blackberries	Sugar-free Bruschetta (see recipe)	Stuffed Goat's Cheese Turkey Burgers (see recipe) served with at least 2 portions of vegetables or a large salad	**Consume up to 2 snacks per day and only when hungry** 10 olives Up to 30g hard cheese 10 Parmesan Crisps with 1 tbsp homemade Guacamole or homemade salsa ½ an avocado topped with balsamic vinegar 50g nuts (not peanuts) 1 Fat Bomb	6–8 glasses of water Tea and coffee (herbal or decaf if you prefer) In coffee and tea, try sticking with double cream or unsweetened almond or coconut milk

Breakfast	Lunch	Dinner	Snacks	Drinks
2 eggs (cooked any way you like), 3 rashers of bacon, 1 good-quality sausage (at least 80% meat), 1 flat mushroom	Large prawn salad: up to 100g prawns with 3 handfuls of salad leaves, 50g cucumber and 8 cherry tomatoes with 2 tbsp olive oil and cider vinegar dressing	Creamy Mushroom and Ham 'Pasta' (see recipe)	**Consume up to 2 snacks per day and only when hungry** 10 olives Up to 30g hard cheese 10 Parmesan Crisps with 1 tbsp homemade Guacamole or homemade salsa ½ an avocado topped with balsamic vinegar 50g nuts (not peanuts) 1 Fat Bomb	6–8 glasses of water Tea and coffee (herbal or decaf if you prefer) In coffee and tea, try sticking with double cream or unsweetened almond or coconut milk

Breakfast	Lunch	Dinner	Snacks	Drinks
Egg, salmon and avocado platter: 3 eggs (cooked any way you like), 50g salmon (any kind) and ½ an avocado	Greek salad: half a cucumber, 10 cherry tomatoes halved, 50g feta cheese with 2–3 tbsp olive oil	Chicken breast stuffed with mozzarella (no more than 50g) wrapped in a slice of Parma ham or bacon then roasted for 20 mins at 180°C, served with 100g steamed green beans and 100g mushrooms cooked in butter	**Consume up to 2 snacks per day and only when hungry** 10 olives Up to 30g hard cheese 10 Parmesan Crisps with 1 tbsp homemade Guacamole or homemade salsa ½ an avocado topped with balsamic vinegar 50g nuts (not peanuts) 1 Fat Bomb	6–8 glasses of water Tea and coffee (herbal or decaf if you prefer) In coffee and tea, try sticking with double cream or unsweetened almond or coconut milk

Breakfast	Lunch	Dinner	Snacks	Drinks
Warm Chia Seed Breakfast Mug (see recipe) topped with 50g berries (optional)	Grilled halloumi salad: up to 60g halloumi cheese with 2 large handfuls of young spinach leaves, 1 handful of rocket, ½ a green pepper, 50g cucumber, with olive oil and cider vinegar dressing (3 parts oil to 1 vinegar)	Spiced omelette: 3 large eggs whisked with 4 tsp double cream, finely chopped onion and red pepper, coriander, cumin and ½–1 tsp chilli powder. Serve with fresh salad or guacamole	**Consume up to 2 snacks per day and only when hungry** 10 olives Up to 30g hard cheese 10 Parmesan Crisps with 1 tbsp homemade Guacamole or homemade salsa ½ an avocado topped with balsamic vinegar 50g nuts (not peanuts) 1 Fat Bomb	6–8 glasses of water Tea and coffee (herbal or decaf if you prefer) In coffee and tea, try sticking with double cream or unsweetened almond or coconut milk

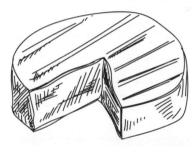

Vegetarian Meal Plan Week 1 and 5

Breakfast	Lunch	Dinner	Snacks	Drinks
3 tbsp natural whole-milk (or Greek) yogurt mixed with 1 tbsp double cream (optional), 1 tbsp coconut flakes, 30g mixed nuts and 50g berries	Green Smoothie (see recipe) with 3 celery stalks and almond butter	Shallow-fried Coconut Camembert (see recipe)	**Consume up to 2 snacks per day and only when hungry** 10 olives Up to 30g hard cheese ½ an avocado topped with balsamic vinegar 50g nuts (not peanuts) 1 Fat Bomb (see recipe)	6–8 glasses of water Tea and coffee (herbal or decaf if you prefer) In coffee and tea, try sticking with double cream or unsweetened almond or coconut milk

Breakfast	Lunch	Dinner	Snacks	Drinks
1 Egg Muffin (see recipe) but substitute the bacon with 150g chopped mushrooms that have been fried for 5 mins in butter)	Grilled halloumi salad: 60g halloumi, 2 large handfuls of young spinach leaves, 1 handful of rocket, ½ a green pepper, 50g cucumber, with olive oil and cider vinegar dressing (3 parts oil to 1 vinegar)	Aubergine 'pizzas': cut aubergine into 1cm discs (up to 8 slices), spread with sundried tomato paste, top with a slice of mozzarella and a slice of Cheddar cheese and sprinkle with basil. Grill for 5–10 minutes. Serve with sautéed spinach	**Consume up to 2 snacks per day and only when hungry** 10 olives Up to 30g hard cheese ½ an avocado topped with balsamic vinegar 50g nuts (not peanuts) 1 Fat Bomb	6–8 glasses of water Tea and coffee (herbal or decaf if you prefer) In coffee and tea, try sticking with double cream or unsweetened almond or coconut milk

Breakfast	Lunch	Dinner	Snacks	Drinks
3 tbsp natural whole-milk (or Greek) yogurt mixed with 1 tbsp double cream (optional), 1 tbsp coconut flakes, 30g mixed nuts and 50g berries	Beetroot and goat's cheese salad: 50g goat's cheese, 50g diced fresh beetroot, 30g walnuts, 2 large handfuls of young spinach leaves, 1 handful of rocket, ½ a green pepper, 50g cucumber, with olive oil and cider vinegar dressing (3 parts oil to 1 vinegar)	Baked Eggs with Asparagus and Mozzarella (see recipe)	**Consume up to 2 snacks per day and only when hungry** 10 olives Up to 30g hard cheese ½ an avocado topped with balsamic vinegar 50g nuts (not peanuts) 1 Fat Bomb	6–8 glasses of water Tea and coffee (herbal or decaf if you prefer) In coffee and tea, try sticking with double cream or unsweetened almond or coconut milk

Breakfast	Lunch	Dinner	Snacks	Drinks
Warm Chia Seed Breakfast Mug (see recipe)	Cherry tomatoes (up to 10) stuffed with soft goat's cheese served with a large salad drizzled with olive oil and cider vinegar	Stuffed Aubergine (see recipe) served on a large bed of spinach	**Consume up to 2 snacks per day and only when hungry** 10 olives Up to 30g hard cheese ½ an avocado topped with balsamic vinegar 50g nuts (not peanuts) 1 Fat Bomb	6–8 glasses of water Tea and coffee (herbal or decaf if you prefer) In coffee and tea, try sticking with double cream or unsweetened almond or coconut milk

Breakfast	Lunch	Dinner	Snacks	Drinks

Breakfast	Lunch	Dinner	Snacks	Drinks
3 tbsp natural whole-milk (or Greek) yogurt mixed with 1 tbsp double cream (optional), 1 tbsp coconut flakes, 30g mixed nuts and 50g berries	Warm goat's cheese salad: up to 60g goat's cheese, grilled and served with 2 large handfuls of young spinach leaves, 1 handful of rocket, ½ a green pepper, 50g cucumber, with olive oil and cider vinegar dressing (3 parts oil to 1 vinegar)	Chargrilled Mediterranean vegetables (aubergine, courgettes, peppers, red onion and tomatoes) and grilled halloumi served on a large bed of spinach sprinkled with walnuts and pumpkin seeds, with olive oil and cider vinegar dressing	**Consume up to 2 snacks per day and only when hungry** 10 olives Up to 30g hard cheese ½ an avocado topped with balsamic vinegar 50g nuts (not peanuts) 1 Fat Bomb	6–8 glasses of water Tea and coffee (herbal or decaf if you prefer) In coffee and tea, try sticking with double cream or unsweetened almond or coconut milk

Breakfast	Lunch	Dinner	Snacks	Drinks
Egg and avocado platter: 3 eggs (cooked any way you like), ½ an avocado and 6 cherry tomatoes	Green Smoothie (see recipe)	2 large flat mushrooms stuffed with mozzarella and ricotta cheese and herbs of your choice, and grilled. Serve with a large salad	**Consume up to 2 snacks per day and only when hungry** 10 olives Up to 30g hard cheese ½ an avocado topped with balsamic vinegar 50g nuts (not peanuts) 1 Fat Bomb	6–8 glasses of water Tea and coffee (herbal or decaf if you prefer) In coffee and tea, try sticking with double cream or unsweetened almond or coconut milk

Breakfast	Lunch	Dinner	Snacks	Drinks
2 tbsp natural whole-milk (or Greek) yogurt mixed with 1 tbsp double cream (optional), 1 tbsp coconut flakes, 30g mixed nuts and 50g berries	Green Smoothie (see recipe)	Cheesy Courgette 'Pasta' (see recipe)	**Consume up to 2 snacks per day and only when hungry** 10 olives Up to 30g hard cheese ½ an avocado topped with balsamic vinegar 50g nuts (not peanuts) 1 Fat Bomb	6–8 glasses of water Tea and coffee (herbal or decaf if you prefer) In coffee and tea, try sticking with double cream or unsweetened almond or coconut milk

6   Low Carb Healthy Fat lifestyle

In this chapter, we are going to take a closer look at what LCHF means and why it may be the best dietary approach for you.

Written with nutritionist Emily Maguire

For this dietary approach to succeed, you need to reappraise old ideas about nutrition. For the past thirty years or more, certain dietary dogmas have shaped our views of nutrition. Many people still believe that eating too much fat will cause weight gain and raise cholesterol, leading to a host of potential health problems. Science and individual experience are now proving that these ideas may not be entirely accurate.

Many people blame themselves when a weight-loss diet doesn't work. Either you didn't try hard enough or there must be something wrong with you. But guess what? Sometimes it really isn't your fault. The key dogma that all you need to do to lose weight is eat a little less and do a little more is flawed: what you eat matters, both for your weight and for your overall health and happiness. Get ready to adopt brand new beliefs and behaviours.

One of the major flaws of conventional nutritional thinking is that the same dietary approach will work for everyone. That every human being on the planet should eat less fat and more carbohydrates. But no two people are exactly the same, so why should we all follow the same pattern of eating?

The LCHF diet that is outlined in this book should be seen as a starting point for you to build on as your body needs. Some people may find that they can tolerate a little more carbohydrate (from certain fruits, and vegetables such as sweet potatoes and pulses), whereas other people will have to be a little stricter: if you experience cravings, mood swings (often caused by intense highs and lows in your blood sugar) or weight gain, you will need to keep your carb intake on the lower side. Similarly, the amount of fat you need will vary from individual to individual. Stick to the portion sizes suggested in this book for at least the first eight weeks of your LCHF lifestyle. In Chapter Thirteen we will take you through the kind of adjustments that you may need to make in the following months. The great thing is that once you reset your body on the LCHF way of eating, it will be able to give off the right signals as to what it needs to remain healthy, signals that will no longer be masked by sugar cravings and unexplainable hunger.

Emily Maguire

My story starts at university, when I was studying for a BSc in Nutrition. The course covered all the standard theories. I was taught that too much fat is bad for you, that the basis of your meals should be carbohydrates and that weight control is all about calories in vs. calories out. In 2008, though, everything that I had thought to be gospel about nutrition was flipped on its head. That was the year I discovered the work of Dr Eric Westman and Dr Will Yancy of Duke University.

It was the summer between the second and third years of my undergrad degree and I had taken some work experience. On the first day, when I found out that I was working at a low-carbohydrate diet company, I came very close to walking out of the building and reporting them for bringing harm to their consumers. I vowed I would stay that day but then not come back. As it turned out, this was the beginning of the end of nutrition as I knew it. That was the first time that I came across the vast amount of science in this field and I was hooked. I had gone down the Alice in Wonderland hole for nutrition and there was no going back.

I spent the final two years of my degree being taught the conventional way while being aware of all of this 'new' information. At the time I was so angry about how nutritionists and dietitians are being taught at degree level. But in a roundabout way I can understand why some people find it hard to accept the notion of low-carbohydrate eating being healthy. If I hadn't stumbled across the science when I did, but had spent four years at university being taught conventionally, then I would now be preaching the low-fat mantra. I am glad that I found the science and went on my own quest to discover the truth.

In 2011, I attended the Nutrition and Metabolism Society symposium in Baltimore and got to meet Professor Richard Feinman, Dr Jeff Volek, Dr Steve Phinney and Dr Eric Westman. I have now completed a world quest where I have shadowed, met with and learnt from some of the top minds within the field of low-carbohydrate nutrition. Many people thought me crazy for packing up my life and making this trip in my own time and without funding. For me, though, this is more than just a job: it is a passion that I will continue to follow and hopefully share with the world.

How LCHF works

The term LCHF stands for Low Carb High Fat, but we prefer to call it Low Carb Healthy Fat. This type of dietary approach has gained much interest over the past few years: you may be familiar with it under names such as the low-carb diet, the ketogenic diet or the Banting diet. While there are slight differences in interpretation, all these diets encapsulate similar nutritional principles.

In simple terms, LCHF is a way of eating that is low in sugars and refined grains while being higher in healthy fats, with an adequate protein intake.

A common belief in conventional nutrition has been that we all need to eat a high amount of carbohydrates as they are essential for energy. While it's true that we do need a certain amount of carbohydrates or sugar, the amount is actually very low. At any one time, for the body to function properly it only requires the equivalent of one teaspoon (5g) of sugar.

That's it! 1 teaspoon is required for normal human life. So to say that half of our energy intake (calories) needs to come from starchy carbohydrates is completely baffling. Some people argue that it is glucose (the type of sugar in our blood) that is essential for energy. It would be more accurate to say that the body prefers to use glucose as its fuel. An essential nutrient is one that the body needs to get from the diet. There are essential fatty acids (fats) and essential amino acids (proteins). These are deemed as essential because the body cannot make them within itself and has to get them from the food we eat. But there are no essential forms of carbohydrates. This means that, if needed, the body can make glucose within itself. As long as your body maintains the 5g of blood sugar that it needs then your body and brain will function well.

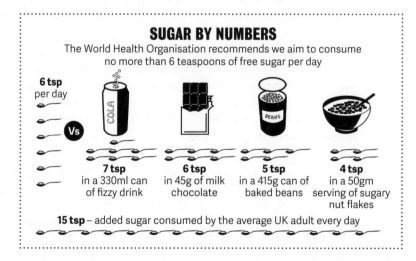

SUGAR BY NUMBERS

The World Health Organisation recommends we aim to consume no more than 6 teaspoons of free sugar per day

6 tsp per day

Vs

7 tsp in a 330ml can of fizzy drink

6 tsp in a 45g of milk chocolate

5 tsp in a 415g can of baked beans

4 tsp in a 50gm serving of sugary nut flakes

15 tsp – added sugar consumed by the average UK adult every day

In fact your body can function on a different type of fuel and this is generally what happens when you follow an LCHF diet. When you restrict your carbohydrates to a certain level it means that your body no longer has enough glucose to use as its preferred fuel, so it must turn to something else instead. The next thing that it turns to is fat. More on this later in the chapter.

In a conventional healthy diet, 50–55% of the calories come from carbohydrates (ideally from whole grains, pulses, vegetables and fruit). If you're eating a standard 2000 calories (kcal) per day, this means about 275g of carbs; if you're following a 1500-calorie weight-loss diet it would be about 200g of carbs. A LCHF diet limits carbohydrates to 5–10% of your daily calorie intake, which means 50g or less of carbs. If you follow the meal plans outlined in this book your carbohydrate intake will be at or below 50g per day.

You may have heard the sayings 'listen to your body' and 'eat until you feel full'. However, when your diet is predominantly based on carbohydrates, especially the refined form, the body's ability to signal satiety is dampened. Once refined carbs are taken out of the diet and replaced with natural, healthy fats, your body's ability to tune into its satiety signals begins operating properly again. In addition, this type of diet in general keeps you feeling fuller and satisfied for longer.

Why follow an LCHF diet?

This dietary approach is not just about weight loss, nor is it a fad diet. When followed correctly, it has been shown to have some extremely beneficial outcomes in a number of areas, including:

- Diabetes
- Metabolic syndrome
- Cardiovascular disease
- Alzheimer's disease
- Epilepsy
- Certain types of cancer
- Skin conditions
- Improvements in mood and cognition
- Reduced cravings
- Improved response to the body's satiety signals

IMPROVEMENT IN BLOOD SUGAR LEVELS

Perhaps one of the most impressive results of adopting the LCHF way of eating is improvements in blood sugar levels. After eating sugary, starchy or refined carbohydrates our blood sugar (glucose) level shoots up and the body has to act quickly to use the energy for storage. Having dramatic spikes and falls in blood sugar throughout the day will cause cravings and increase hunger. Scientists are increasingly finding that high blood sugar levels are at the core of many conditions, such as diabetes, with emerging evidence linking it to Alzheimer's disease. Stability in blood sugar levels will also result in an improvement in mood and cognition.

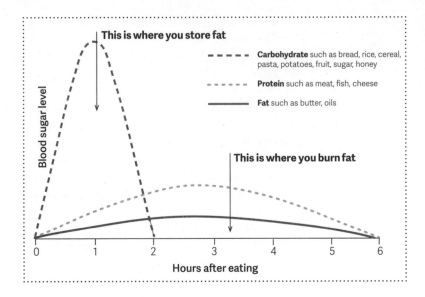

This is where you store fat

- - - - **Carbohydrate** such as bread, rice, cereal, pasta, potatoes, fruit, sugar, honey

· · · · · **Protein** such as meat, fish, cheese

——— **Fat** such as butter, oils

This is where you burn fat

Blood sugar level

Hours after eating

The LCHF diet and ketosis

Simply put, ketosis is when the body will burn fat to give it energy. Carbohydrates are broken down in the body to produce a simple sugar known as glucose. Under normal conditions, your body will burn this for energy. When you restrict your carbohydrates to 50g per day or less, your body can no longer get the energy it needs from this amount of carbohydrates. It then needs to bring in other mechanisms and fuels in order to function. This is where fat comes in. The body can get the energy it needs from stored fat and the fat content within food.

When you restrict carbohydrates in your diet to less than 50g per day, your body will automatically turn to its stored form of glucose, known as glycogen. Glycogen is stored in the liver and the muscles; this is how the body stores excess glucose eaten in the diet. However,

the body has a very small storage capacity for glucose – about 300–400g – with any excess then being stored as fat. This amount of glucose will only be able to provide the body with energy for around 12–24 hours. Once the body has used all of this up, it starts looking for other sources to give it energy – enter gluconeogenesis. This simply means the body's ability to make glucose out of non-glucose molecules. Even more simply put, it means that the body can take fat and protein and turn it into glucose. After the glycogen store has been used up, the body will switch to gluconeogenesis to start getting the energy that it needs. This process is something that happens to most of us when we are sleeping and is one of the body's many survival mechanisms to cope with times without food. Once the body realises that you aren't going to be feeding it the quick-releasing energy of glucose, it looks for another source of energy. This is where ketosis (the process of burning fat) comes into play, and this is the principle behind the ketogenic diet.

Calories in vs. calories out

Many people still believe that the only successful way to lose weight is simply to eat less and move more. We now know that the quality of food matters just as much as the quantity. Having a diet that is based predominantly on sugar and refined grains can mask the body's natural ability to signal when it is full. Even worse, many processed foods have been deliberately created to mask your normal satiety signals. Food manufacturers actually hire food scientists to come up with just the right formula of fat + sugar + salt to equal tricking your body into thinking that you aren't full. This is why it seems as though you can eat an abundance of junk food without ever really feeling full, or having a very short-term satiety. Once you remove sugar and refined grains from your diet and instead fill up on healthy fats, you allow your body to naturally reset so that it can send the appropriate satiety signals.

That being said, it is a mistake to think that when you are following an LCHF template you do not need to worry about your calorie intake. While it is true that you don't necessarily need to count calories in vs. calories out in the conventional way, that is not to say that calories themselves do not mean anything. If you are someone who needs to lose weight then having an excess of calories, particularly from fat, can still hinder your progress.

When your body burns fat to provide energy, ketone bodies, or ketones, are released as a by-product. Ketone bodies can be measured in the urine, blood or breath.

A high ketone reading (particularly in the blood) simply shows that the body is burning fat for energy. It doesn't show exactly where this fat is coming from. If you are ingesting a lot of calories from fat, particularly liquid fat (coconut oil, cream in your coffee), then your body will more than likely burn that fat before burning body fat. So a high ketone reading does not necessarily mean fat loss from your body. There is a huge difference between fat burning and weight loss.

Ketogenic vs. non-ketogenic LCHF

As we have said, there is some flexibility within the LCHF diet: different people have different needs, and the exact intake of carbohydrate, fat and protein will vary from day to day. For some people it is not necessary to maintain a ketogenic state where they limit themselves to a maximum of 50g of carbohydrates a day. For individuals who are looking to lose weight or have consistently high blood sugar levels, we recommend that they stay below 50g of carbohydrates. However, people who are fairly active or who don't have blood sugar problems may be able to cope with a higher carbohydrate intake – up to a maximum of 120g per day. What is important is that the source of carbohydrates will never be sugar or refined carbohydrates; instead it will be in the form of whole foods such as vegetables, pulses and fruits.

A family affair

Can your children safely join you on a LCHF diet, devoid of starches and whole grains? The time constraints on modern lives means it's impossible to cook separate dinners for each family member. If the rest of your family don't do it, chances are, neither will you. Plus, if carbs and sugar are in the house, your willpower may not be strong enough to stay away from those tempting foods. Your success may depend on the whole family eating Low Carb High Fat

★

Tips for making the transition to Sugar Free kids

1. TALK TO YOUR KIDS
Young children may not be able to understand the science but they can learn which foods make their brains and bodies grow healthy and strong.

2. INVOLVE YOUR CHILDREN
Let your children have some say in grocery shopping, food preparation and meal planning.

3. GROW YOUR OWN VEGGIES AND HERBS
From lettuce and spinach to parsley, add it to your meals.

4. CREATE BOUNDARIES BY IDENTIFYING A SET TIME AND PLACE FOR MEALTIMES
Eat together as a family, creating happy meals and family time together.

5. GIVE CHOICES WITHIN REASON
Offer two healthy options, giving your children the opportunity to choose. This stops them from feeling that they've been forced to comply.

6. DON'T GIVE IN WHEN THEY CRAVE JUNK AT HOME
By doing this you're doing them a great disservice. Strive for your kids to eat healthily 80 per cent of the time.

7. USE SUGAR-FREE OR CARB-FREE VERSIONS OF THEIR FAVOURITE FOOD
There are many resources online once you start looking.

8. PACK INTERESTING AND COLOURFUL LUNCHBOXES
Keep your kids' food choices fun, fresh and inviting. See page 131 for some ideas.

Karen

I run a Sugar Free house, meaning there are no sugar-laden, junk-filled foods or beverages in my house. We eat whole foods (meat, vegetables and some fruits) and we stick to food as close to its original form as possible. Let's face it . . . sugar and processed carbs have no nutritional value. We drink water, tea and coffee (with whole milk or cream). The transition for my family was challenging at first, but it took only a couple of weeks for us to settle into our new, calmer, Sugar Free household routine.

During the transition I faced a dilemma. Logically it made sense, but emotionally and psychologically I worried 'Am I doing them harm by not allowing them to have sugar?' and 'Could this create an eating disorder in my children?' The answer to all these questions remains no. I stand firm in my belief that I'm not doing my children harm by providing them with nutritious meals and snacks.

As strict as I am at home though, I allow my kids to make their own choices when we're out. When at kids' parties, out for dinner or lunch or at school events my kids can choose to eat whatever they want. At first they gravitated to junk, sweets and processed foods but they soon realised for themselves the effect it had on their bodies. My oldest son has never been able to handle the effects of sugar very well. He turns into a Duracell bunny, unable to listen or cooperate much. We started referring to this behaviour as the 'sugar monster' being unleashed in him. It's not deemed as good or bad. Sugar definitely affects his behaviour and moods.

Even though I'm vigilant about what I fill my Sugar Free space with, this does not mean a tray of choc-chip muffins won't occasionally sneak into the kitchen. That, however, is the exception to the rule.

I have found what works for me and believe it's up to every one of us to make our own decisions and lead by example.

9. TURN TRADITIONAL SUGAR AND CARB-FILLED FOODS INTO SUGAR-FREE DELIGHTS
Try these ideas:

● Make chocolate-chip muffins using almond flour or coconut flour and 70% cocoa solids dark chocolate.

● Modify pancakes using nut flour or coconut flour.

● Make crisps and chips at home using root veg such as sweet potatoes, carrots and beetroot.

Lisa's story

I first went on a diet in 1991 when I got married. I was not overweight; I just thought this was what brides-to-be did. After marriage I gained weight gradually – I blamed my four pregnancies. But the truth is that after I'd lived through a number of traumas food became my faithful friend. I saw a caption in a magazine asking if I was addicted to sugar. My first thought was 'I am not!' But I took the quiz and ticked eleven of thirteen questions. By this time I'd tried every possible diet, injection, tablet, protein and shake. Through the magazine article I contacted Karen Thomson about the HELP Program. I was desperate. The scary part was it promised not a diet but a commitment to a lifestyle.

With the support of the programme, I discovered I am an addict. That was always a title reserved for people with no self-control, whose lives were out of control. My addiction was just not obvious to me. Like a smoker I lied to myself – I ate because I liked good food and could diet and lose the weight whenever I wanted to . . . Like smokers who just smoke because they 'like it' who insist they can 'quit' whenever they want to. The lies are a lot easier than having to deal with the addiction.

Now LCHF has become my way of life. I haven't dieted for over fifteen months and I've lost 24kg. I've learnt that I am enough; that I have all I need inside of me and not inside the fridge. I feel healthy and food is not a punishment or a reward but something I use to nourish my body. Food keeps my engine running and I'm no longer inviting illness and obesity into my space. I've gone from a size 20 to a healthy size 12. My body shape has changed, my clothes fit differently; I'm free to buy from any shop I like. I don't have to start looking at the back of the rail. I don't have to disguise a bloated tummy, love handles, tuckshop upper arms, chicken wing underarms . . . I feel completely free to express myself through how I present myself from the inside out.

It's not always plain sailing. Although I have not deliberately had sugar since January 2013, I have polished off a packet of Doritos many times. I recently went to a dinner where they were serving filo pastry with cheese and a garnish of preserved fig. I thought I could have just one. Then the sweetness triggered something deep down and I had six or more . . . I was completely unable to control myself. I've realised I have to stay away from anything remotely sweet.

I have my health back. I feel worthwhile. I'm living my life making choices every day that are first in my interest, and then for the benefit of my husband and four beautiful children. When I'm happy and in charge of me, our family works better.

I've started running and I love who it makes me. I did my first half-marathon in 2014 after forty-five years of little to no exercise. It is a big deal and has motivated many of my friends and family to start walking, running, jogging and moving.

I love getting up, dressing up and showing up in the mornings. Going out at night is easy now, no matter the occasion, because I feel like I'm my best self and I did this for me. My husband quite fancies my new look. He tells me and I overhear him telling others.

WEEKLY JOURNAL EXERCISE

Take a few minutes to reflect on your week and this stage of your journey:

1 What were your greatest successes this week?
2 How will you build on your successes?
3 Did you stick to your meal plan?
4 Did you maintain abstinence from sugar and carbs?
5 If not, what triggered you to relapse or slip?
   What have you learnt from this experience?
6 What exercise did you do this week?
7 Are you unhappy about anything that happened this week?
8 Have you been affirming yourself?
9 What will you do differently next week to support your journey in recovery positively?
10 Make a list of ten things you are grateful for.

♥
Affirmation
I deserve
great health.

DAY 8

Breakfast	Lunch	Dinner	Snacks	Drinks
Green Smoothie (see recipe)	3 scrambled eggs with ham, ¼ of a courgette and 6 cherry tomatoes	Chicken Aubergine Lasagne (see recipe; keep some for tomorrow) served with a green salad dressed with olive oil	**Consume up to 2 snacks per day and only when hungry** 10 olives Up to 30g hard cheese 10 Parmesan Crisps with 1 tbsp homemade Guacamole or homemade salsa ½ an avocado topped with balsamic vinegar 50g nuts (not peanuts) 1 Fat Bomb	6–8 glasses of water Tea and coffee (herbal or decaf if you prefer) In coffee and tea, try sticking with double cream or unsweetened almond or coconut milk

DAY 9

Breakfast	Lunch	Dinner	Snacks	Drinks
Greek-style omelette made with 3 eggs, 40g feta cheese, 1 tsp dried basil and ½ tsp dried oregano 10 olives and 6 cherry tomatoes topped with fresh coriander	Creamy Avocado Soup (see recipe) with 1 or 2 Seed Crackers (see recipe)	Chicken Aubergine Lasagne (left over from last night's dinner) served with a green salad dressed with olive oil	**Consume up to 2 snacks per day and only when hungry** 10 olives Up to 30g hard cheese 10 Parmesan Crisps with 1 tbsp homemade Guacamole or homemade salsa ½ an avocado topped with balsamic vinegar 50g nuts (not peanuts) 1 Fat Bomb	6–8 glasses of water Tea and coffee (herbal or decaf if you prefer) In coffee and tea, try sticking with double cream or unsweetened almond or coconut milk

DAY 10

Breakfast	Lunch	Dinner	Snacks	Drinks
3 tbsp natural whole-milk (or Greek) yogurt mixed with 1 tbsp double cream (optional), 1 tbsp coconut flakes, 30g mixed nuts and 50g berries	Spiced omelette: 3 large eggs whisked with 4 tsp milk or double cream, finely chopped onion and red pepper, coriander, cumin and ½–1 tsp chilli powder. Serve with fresh salad or guacamole	Chilli Con Carne (see recipe; keep some for tomorrow) with Cauliflower Rice (see recipe)	**Consume up to 2 snacks per day and only when hungry** 10 olives Up to 30g hard cheese 10 Parmesan Crisps with 1 tbsp homemade Guacamole or homemade salsa ½ an avocado topped with balsamic vinegar 50g nuts (not peanuts) 1 Fat Bomb	6–8 glasses of water Tea and coffee (herbal or decaf if you prefer) In coffee and tea, try sticking with double cream or unsweetened almond or coconut milk

Breakfast	Lunch	Dinner	Snacks	Drinks
3 rashers of bacon with 50g cream cheese and 50g berries	Caprese Salad (see recipe)	Chilli Con Carne (left over from last night's dinner) with Cauliflower Rice	**Consume up to 2 snacks per day and only when hungry** 10 olives Up to 30g hard cheese 10 Parmesan Crisps with 1 tbsp homemade Guacamole or homemade salsa ½ an avocado topped with balsamic vinegar 50g nuts (not peanuts) 1 Fat Bomb	6–8 glasses of water Tea and coffee (herbal or decaf if you prefer) In coffee and tea, try sticking with double cream or unsweetened almond or coconut milk

Breakfast	Lunch	Dinner	Snacks	Drinks
3 tbsp natural whole-milk (or Greek) yogurt mixed with (50g) sugar-free granola and 50g berries	Chicken and bacon salad: up to 100g chicken and 50g bacon with 3 handfuls of salad leaves, 50g cucumber and 8 cherry tomatoes, with olive oil and cider vinegar dressing	Salmon fillet (grilled, baked or fried) topped with 1 tbsp homemade Green Pesto (see recipe), served with 3 grilled vine tomatoes and 8 spears of asparagus (served with butter)	**Consume up to 2 snacks per day and only when hungry** 10 olives Up to 30g hard cheese 10 Parmesan Crisps with 1 tbsp homemade Guacamole or homemade salsa ½ an avocado topped with balsamic vinegar 50g nuts (not peanuts) 1 Fat Bomb	6–8 glasses of water Tea and coffee (herbal or decaf if you prefer) In coffee and tea, try sticking with double cream or unsweetened almond or coconut milk

Breakfast	Lunch	Dinner	Snacks	Drinks
2 eggs (cooked any way you like), 3 rashers of bacon, 1 good-quality sausage (at least 80% meat), 1 flat mushroom	Thai Green Curry (see recipe)	2 grilled lamb chops served with 2 portions of vegetables	**Consume up to 2 snacks per day and only when hungry** 10 olives Up to 30g hard cheese 10 Parmesan Crisps with 1 tbsp homemade Guacamole or homemade salsa ½ an avocado topped with balsamic vinegar 50g nuts (not peanuts) 1 Fat Bomb	6–8 glasses of water Tea and coffee (herbal or decaf if you prefer) In coffee and tea, try sticking with double cream or unsweetened almond or coconut milk

Breakfast	Lunch	Dinner	Snacks	Drinks
2 Egg and Parma Ham Cups (see recipe) served with 1 tbsp sour cream	Super Green Soup (see recipe) served with 1 slice Nut and Seed Loaf	1 medium-steak (about 150g) with garlic butter and roasted celeriac (50g uncooked weight) and sweet potato chips (50g uncooked weight)	**Consume up to 2 snacks per day and only when hungry** 10 olives Up to 30g hard cheese 10 Parmesan Crisps with 1 tbsp homemade Guacamole or homemade salsa ½ an avocado topped with balsamic vinegar 50g nuts (not peanuts) 1 Fat Bomb	6–8 glasses of water Tea and coffee (herbal or decaf if you prefer) In coffee and tea, try sticking with double cream or unsweetened almond or coconut milk

Breakfast	Lunch	Dinner	Snacks	Drinks
3 tbsp natural whole-milk (or Greek) yogurt mixed with 50g sugar-free Nut Granola (see recipe)	Warm goat's cheese and walnut salad: 50g goat's cheese (heated under the grill for 5 minutes), 30g walnuts, 2 large handfuls of young spinach leaves, 1 handful of rocket, ½ a green pepper, 50g cucumber, with olive oil and cider vinegar dressing (3 parts oil to 1 vinegar)	2 slices of low-carb pizza, served with Celeriac Chips (see recipe)	**Consume up to 2 snacks per day and only when hungry** 10 olives Up to 30g hard cheese ½ an avocado topped with balsamic vinegar 50g nuts (not peanuts) 1 Fat Bomb	6–8 glasses of water Tea and coffee (herbal or decaf if you prefer) In coffee and tea, try sticking with double cream or unsweetened almond or coconut milk

Breakfast	Lunch	Dinner	Snacks	Drinks
Egg 'muffins': whisk together 4 eggs, chopped tomato, green pepper and onion. Pour into buttered muffin tins and fill halfway. Bake in the oven at 160°C for 15 minutes or until cooked	Grilled halloumi salad: 60g halloumi, 2 large handfuls of young spinach leaves, 1 handful of rocket, ½ a green pepper, 50g cucumber, with olive oil and cider vinegar dressing (3 parts oil to 1 vinegar)	Aubergine 'pizzas': cut aubergine into 1cm discs (up to 8 slices), spread with sundried tomato paste, top with a slice of mozzarella and a slice of Cheddar cheese and sprinkle with basil. Grill for 5–10 minutes. Serve with sautéed spinach	**Consume up to 2 snacks per day and only when hungry** 10 olives Up to 30g hard cheese ½ an avocado topped with balsamic vinegar 50g nuts (not peanuts) 1 Fat Bomb	6–8 glasses of water Tea and coffee (herbal or decaf if you prefer) In coffee and tea, try sticking with double cream or unsweetened almond or coconut milk

Breakfast	Lunch	Dinner	Snacks	Drinks
Warm Chia Seed Breakfast Mug (see recipe)	Beetroot and goat's cheese salad: 50g goat's cheese, 50g diced fresh beetroot, 30g walnuts, 2 large handfuls of young spinach leaves, 1 handful of rocket, ½ a green pepper, 50g cucumber, with olive oil and cider vinegar dressing (3 parts oil to 1 vinegar)	Mushroom Stroganoff (see recipe and keep some for tomorrow) with Cauliflower Rice (see recipe)	**Consume up to 2 snacks per day and only when hungry** 10 olives Up to 30g hard cheese ½ an avocado topped with balsamic vinegar 50g nuts (not peanuts) 1 Fat Bomb	6–8 glasses of water Tea and coffee (herbal or decaf if you prefer) In coffee and tea, try sticking with double cream or unsweetened almond or coconut milk

Breakfast	Lunch	Dinner	Snacks	Drinks
Egg and avocado platter: 3 eggs (cooked any way you like), ½ an avocado and 6 cherry tomatoes	2 slices of low-carb Vegetarian Pizza (see recipe) with a large salad	Mushroom Stroganoff (left over from last night's dinner) with Cauliflower Rice	**Consume up to 2 snacks per day and only when hungry** 10 olives Up to 30g hard cheese ½ an avocado topped with balsamic vinegar 50g nuts (not peanuts) 1 Fat Bomb	6–8 glasses of water Tea and coffee (herbal or decaf if you prefer) In coffee and tea, try sticking with double cream or unsweetened almond or coconut milk

Breakfast	Lunch	Dinner	Snacks	Drinks
3 tbsp natural whole-milk (or Greek) yogurt with 50g of sugar-free Nut Granola (see recipe)	Grilled halloumi salad: up to 60g halloumi, 2 large handfuls of young spinach leaves, 1 handful of rocket, ½ a green pepper, 50g cucumber, with olive oil and cider vinegar dressing (3 parts oil to 1 vinegar)	Spinach and Courgette Burgers (see recipe) topped with Cheddar cheese and served with a large salad drizzled with olive oil	**Consume up to 2 snacks per day and only when hungry** 10 olives Up to 30g hard cheese ½ an avocado topped with balsamic vinegar 50g nuts (not peanuts) 1 Fat Bomb	6–8 glasses of water Tea and coffee (herbal or decaf if you prefer) In coffee and tea, try sticking with double cream or unsweetened almond or coconut milk

Breakfast	Lunch	Dinner	Snacks	Drinks
Egg and avocado platter: 3 eggs (cooked any way you like) and ½ an avocado (those not as sensitive to sugar can add 6 cherry tomatoes)	Green Soup (see recipe)	Cauliflower Mac 'n' Cheese Bake (see recipe) served with a large salad dressed with olive oil	**Consume up to 2 snacks per day and only when hungry** 10 olives Up to 30g hard cheese ½ an avocado topped with balsamic vinegar 50g nuts (not peanuts) 1 Fat Bomb	6–8 glasses of water Tea and coffee (herbal or decaf if you prefer) In coffee and tea, try sticking with double cream or unsweetened almond or coconut milk

Breakfast	Lunch	Dinner	Snacks	Drinks
3 tbsp natural whole-milk (or Greek) yogurt mixed with 1 tbsp double cream (optional), 1 tbsp coconut flakes, 30g mixed nuts and 50g berries	1 Mocha Protein Smoothie (see recipe)	Stuffed Aubergine (see recipe)	**Consume up to 2 snacks per day and only when hungry** 10 olives Up to 30g hard cheese ½ an avocado topped with balsamic vinegar 50g nuts (not peanuts) 1 Fat Bomb	6–8 glasses of water Tea and coffee (herbal or decaf if you prefer) In coffee and tea, try sticking with double cream or unsweetened almond or coconut milk

USEFUL RESOURCES

Try these websites for advice and inspiring stories about LCHF eating:

- dietdoctor.com
- lowcarbgenesis.com
- hemsleyandhemsley.com
- livinlavidalowcarb.com
- authoritynutrition.com

Another handy reference is *The Real Meal Revolution: The Radical, Sustainable Approach to Healthy Eating* by Professor Tim Noakes, Jonno Proudfoot and Sally-Ann Creed (Robinson, 2015).

Who am I?

You've taken the first steps in creating a new healthy life for yourself, but where are you going? Do you see yourself as a healthy, mindful and energetic person? In Week Three I'm introducing you to your addict self and helping you create a future vision for yourself.

Your addict self

Addiction can be described as a downward spiral of destructive behaviours that rob us of self-esteem, self-worth and self-love. It's a misguided attempt to avoid pain or even experience happiness. Very simply put, addiction refers to the compulsive pursuit of a substance or behaviour despite the negative consequences. Through addiction our inner lives (thoughts, feelings and beliefs) and outer lives (actions and behaviours) become restricted and we lose our freedom.

As sugar and carb addicts we indulge in unhealthy forms of dependence on sugar and carbohydrates to change or suppress the way we feel. We also use the object of our addiction to soothe ourselves, and very likely

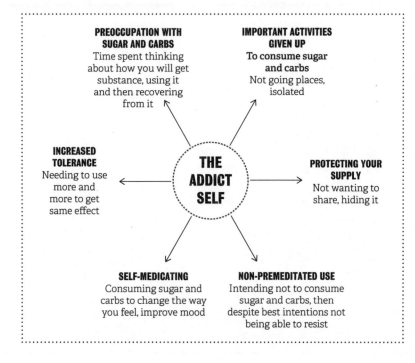

PREOCCUPATION WITH SUGAR AND CARBS
Time spent thinking about how you will get substance, using it and then recovering from it

IMPORTANT ACTIVITIES GIVEN UP
To consume sugar and carbs
Not going places, isolated

INCREASED TOLERANCE
Needing to use more and more to get same effect

THE ADDICT SELF

PROTECTING YOUR SUPPLY
Not wanting to share, hiding it

SELF-MEDICATING
Consuming sugar and carbs to change the way you feel, improve mood

NON-PREMEDITATED USE
Intending not to consume sugar and carbs, then despite best intentions not being able to resist

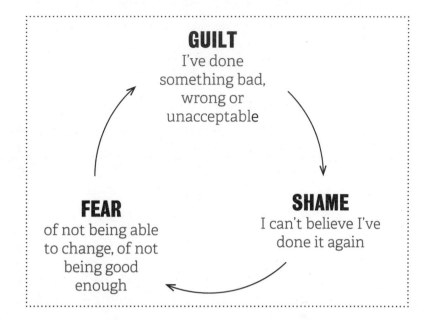

GUILT
I've done something bad, wrong or unacceptable

SHAME
I can't believe I've done it again

FEAR
of not being able to change, of not being good enough

use it to deny our own needs. We can end up feeling hopeless, lost and alone. We often believe this to be our true identity, feeling there is little hope for change.

While in an addictive cycle most of us are motivated by three emotions: guilt, shame and fear.

These feelings feed each other; they are debilitating and create a vicious cycle.

Guilt, fear and shame create negative core beliefs within us about who we are and what we can or can't become – in other words, our addict self. If internalised and left unresolved, these feelings take over and plunge us deeper into our downward spiral. But addiction is not our identity and we are not alone. We may have been indulging in addictive behaviours but that is not who we are.

A life in recovery from addiction can be described as an upward spiral into widening circles of self-love, freedom and connection to your authentic self. By connecting with your authentic self you're able to 'marry' your inner life (feelings and beliefs) with your outer life (behaviour and actions) to create fulfilment.

Karen

I remember the first time I admitted to myself that I was addicted to sugar and carbs. Deep down I knew this was the truth, but my mind kept trying to convince me I was insane to feel that way. I had to take a good look at my behaviour surrounding sugar and carbs – it didn't take me long to realise that I was out of control. By admitting I am a sugar and a carb addict I've given myself permission to start my recovery process. But I also realise I am not my addict self, I'm so much more than that.

JOURNAL EXERCISE

One of the first steps in recovery from sugar and carb addiction is admitting you are an addict, and that your life has become unmanageable due to thoughts, feelings, behaviour and actions being bent on destruction.

Can you identify with any of the following addictive behaviours?
- Obsessive thoughts about sugar and carbs
- Dishonesty about your consumption of sugar and carbs (such as quantities)
- Manipulation
- Shame and guilt after eating or bingeing
- Preoccupation with body image
- Restricting activities due to weight and/or eating habits
- Sugar and carbs used for nurturing or rewards
- Low self-esteem based on weight control and control of eating
- Fantasies about a better life when you're thin
- Feeling tormented by your eating habits
- Despair
- Sadness
- Feeling lost and alone
- Eating in secret
- Once you start eating sugar you cannot stop

Even though you may be able to identify with many of the above statements, it's important to remember these do not define you. This is not how you need to live the rest of your life.

A life in recovery can mean living a life you may think unobtainable. Letting go of your sugar and carb addiction can feel similar to ending a relationship with your best friend. Giving up familiar coping mechanisms or addictive behaviours can feel incredibly scary and uncomfortable, as can taking responsibility for our health and our selves. One of the greatest gifts of recovery is that we get to know and build a new relationship with ourselves, and it can be defined in any way. Are you ready to start defining a new life for yourself?

Journal exercise

Take a few moments to reflect about when you've been successful. What do you think helped? Now think about all the successful people you know, whether it's a parent, businesswoman, leader or student. What makes them successful?

Understanding success

We believe successful people embody the following characteristics:

1

Focus – ability to concentrate and ignore distractions

2

Persistence – able to go after their goal despite obstacles or rejection

3

Vision – of who they are and where they want to go

4

Inquiry – ability to continually ask questions not only of people around them, but of themselves

As successful addicts we already have these things in abundance:

1

Focus – when craving sugar or carbohydrates, it's the only thing you can focus on; nothing else matters

2

Persistence – nothing will stand in the way of satisfying that craving

3

Vision – your mind has a clear picture of what will satisfy that craving

4

Inquiry – where will you find satisfaction for that craving?

So that was a little bit tongue in cheek, but it illustrates that you already have what it takes to be successful:

1

Focus – on your recovery (not your addiction)

2

Persistence – even if you relapse, keep the bigger picture in mind

3

Vision – what is your vision for yourself?

4

Inquiry – what can you do right now for recovery? how can you learn from others? what support do you need?

Journal exercise

Take a few moments to reflect on other questions to ask about your sugar and carb addiction recovery.

Creating a vision for yourself

In this section we're going to focus on your vision of yourself. Who is the healthy you? What about the successful you? The two journal exercises on the next page will help you explore this. The first exercise is writing a story, while the second is creating a Vision Story for yourself. Do the one that most appeals (or do both).

Karen

Every year on New Year's Eve I invite family members and friends (including the kids) to get together for a little ceremony. We do a short guided meditation, focusing on visualising what we'd like to attract into our lives. We then sit together at the dining room table with piles of magazines, crayons, scissors, cardboard and glue, and we create our magical vision boards for the year ahead. I stick my vision board in my office and look at it daily, affirming myself that I deserve the best. I believe if I focus on something it will grow.

JOURNAL EXERCISE
Vision exercise one – write a story (20–30 minutes)

Find a quiet place where you can sit undisturbed with your journal. Take a deep breath and project yourself five years into the future. Think about a healthy you, free from sugar and carb addiction, and living a successful, fulfilled life. Now write a story based on this life. Use these questions as a guideline:

1 What does my physical space look like? Where do I live? What does my furniture look like? How do I dress? What's in my wardrobe?
2 Am I working? What kind of work am I doing? What are my colleagues like?
3 How am I spending my spare time? What activities do I participate in that refresh and lift my soul?
4 What are my relationships like – romantic, family, friends and colleagues?
5 What exercise am I doing?
6 How do I feel inside? What emotions surface when I imagine this future self?
7 As a healthy, energetic person, what are my dreams and goals?

JOURNAL EXERCISE

Vision exercise two – create a Vision Story (30–45 minutes)

For this exercise you'll need a large piece of cardboard, at least five magazines, scissors and glue. When you're ready, take a deep breath and project yourself five years into the future. Think about a healthy you, free from sugar and carb addiction, and living a successful, fulfilled life.

Spend 15–20 minutes paging through the magazines. Rip out pages with images or words that appeal to you. Don't think about why; just tear them out. Now cut out the images or words from those ripped-out pages. Take them and create a collage on your piece of cardboard – your Vision Story. A good tip is to lay the images on the cardboard before sticking them down. You can move images around, overlay them with words and group similar images or themes together. When you're happy with your Vision Story – remember this represents the future you – stick the images onto the cardboard.

Display the board in a place where you can see it every day.

★

Tips for managing emotional cravings for sugar and carbs

We're so used to using sugar and carbs to deal with difficult situations and suppress challenging emotions. Managing these situations and emotions without food or eating can be a frightening prospect. When you first give up sugar and carbs and start living a life in recovery it's completely normal to crave your 'comfort' foods. It sometimes feels as though you have a hollow inside, and that only by indulging in your comfort foods will you fill it. Take a deep breath and return to Week One, and the list of coping activities you created to help deal with your emotions. Identify one or two that could help you during your craving moments. It's important to try to identify the feeling that needs to be soothed.

Another trick is to eat a teaspoonful of fat such as coconut oil. This should take care of that physical craving.

Karen

When I first gave up sugar and carbs I was surprised at the intensity of my cravings. It was hard to distinguish between emotional and physical cravings, so I made sure I took care of both. I'd eat a teaspoon of coconut oil, which took care of the physical craving, and I'd also get active. I spent a lot of time walking around the block, but it worked and I didn't end up feeding my addict with food.

Hannah's story

I was put on slimming tablets when I was eleven and this was the start of my eating disorder. I became obsessed with being thin.

At sixteen I started gaining weight after a traumatic event. I turned to food for comfort. I remained overweight and continued overeating until I was nineteen, and started restricting again. I used laxatives and ate as little as possible until I was hospitalised for anorexia with my weight dangerously low. I also started drinking and smoking and quickly became addicted to both substances.

I remained underweight and continued with the same eating pattern until I was thirty, when I started comfort eating again. I gained a massive amount of weight.

My journey to recovery began when I was thirty-five. Not only was I dealing with an eating disorder but also co-dependency, alcohol, nicotine and prescription medication addiction.

Only in my forties did I start the LCHF way of eating. I joined a challenge which was to follow the LCHF way of eating and enter into a general lifestyle change. I was initially focused on losing weight. The more information I gathered the more I realised that it was not a weight-loss programme but rather a lifestyle choice. I've been inspired by others who are on the programme. I have seen how this programme has changed their relationship with themselves.

→

For me abstinence is not eating or drinking refined carbohydrates and sugar. I also only eat when I'm hungry. Due to my history of anorexia, however, I do have to monitor this closely as restricting can become a primary motivation.

Recovery is a process of self-care in all areas of my life. Spiritually, mentally, emotionally and of course physically. Regular prayer and meditation and practising gratitude every day is part of my spiritual and emotional care. Also being of service to others and accessing support. For mental, emotional and spiritual care I see a therapist and work the twelve-step programme. I also attend support groups.

Getting enough exercise but keeping a balance by getting enough rest is very important and it's something I strive towards. I also try to have fun now and again.

I was recently seriously ill and was hospitalised. I did not have the strength or presence of mind to be vigilant, and also due to a lack of choice I ate bread, rice and sugar. I also ate fruit. When I left the hospital I was able to abstain from the bread and rice right away but could not control the sugar cravings. I could not understand why the cravings did not abate as I was not eating sugar. I eventually realised my problem was fruit. I had continued to eat fruit because I had heard other people say that they ate fruit. Once I stopped eating the fruit my sugar cravings stopped.

The benefits of changing my lifestyle have been profound. I shed weight (a total of 35kg). I was also able to let go of other aspects of my life that were holding me back. I never felt good enough or able to do certain things. I never expected to be treated with respect, as I did not respect myself and my own body. While in the process of losing the weight I filed for divorce from an abusive partner and I have been promoted at work. I have formed some good friendships and most importantly have a loving and caring relationship with myself. Not only do I think I'm good enough, I think I'm fabulous. My future looks exciting and I know if I stay on this path, striving for progress and not perfection, I will achieve my goals, one at a time.

WEEKLY JOURNAL EXERCISE

Take a few minutes to reflect on your week and this stage of your journey:

1. What were your greatest successes this week?
2. How will you build on your successes?
3. Did you stick to your meal plan?
4. Did you maintain abstinence from sugar and carbs?
5. If not, what triggered you to relapse or slip?
   What have you learnt from this experience?
6. What exercise did you do this week?
7. Are you unhappy about anything that happened this week?
8. Have you been affirming yourself?
9. What will you do differently next week to support your journey in recovery positively?
10. Make a list of ten things you are grateful for.

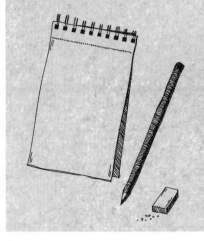

Affirmation

Today I love
and accept
myself
exactly as
I am.

21-day check-in

At the beginning of Week One we gave you a few basic measures we thought would be helpful in tracking your progress. Completing Week Three ends the 21-day challenge. Take some time to record these measurements now:

MEASUREMENT	BEGINNING WEEK ONE	21 DAYS	END OF WEEK EIGHT
Weigh yourself. At the gym, at the doctor or at home.			
Take your waist measurement. This is the narrowest point on your torso.			
Take your hip measurement. Feel for your hipbones and measure across the widest part.			
(If female) Take your bust measurement. Take two measurements: under your bust and across your breasts.			
What are your overall energy levels? Rate out of 10 (0 is no energy and 10 is on top of the world).			
What is your mood generally? Mostly irritable and annoyed? Do you look forward to the day or feel grumpy when you wake up? Reflect on this in your journal.			

USEFUL RESOURCES

Check out the informative blog entries and videos from Donna Margaret McCallum, aka the 'Fairy Godmother'.

For instance, her Goal Setting and Dream Mapping section has an audio-downloadable programme to help you focus on your dreams and goals, with action steps to turn them into reality. See fairygodmotherinc.com

Martha Beck's *Finding Your Own North Star: Claiming the Life You Were Meant to Live* (Piatkus Books, 2001) is a practical guide to help you find what you want in life and live more joyfully.

DAY 15

Breakfast	Lunch	Dinner	Snacks	Drinks
3 tbsp natural whole-milk yogurt with 50g of sugar-free Nut Granola (see recipe)	Salmon (100–120g uncooked) fillet, baked or grilled, with 1 tbsp homemade pesto, served with 2 portions of vegetables	Philly Cheese Steak Stuffed Mushrooms (see recipe) with a large side salad	**Consume up to 2 snacks per day and only when hungry** 10 olives Up to 30g hard cheese 10 Parmesan Crisps with 1 tbsp homemade Guacamole or homemade salsa ½ an avocado topped with balsamic vinegar 50g nuts (not peanuts) 1 Fat Bomb	6–8 glasses of water Tea and coffee (herbal or decaf if you prefer) In coffee and tea, try sticking with double cream or unsweetened almond or coconut milk

DAY 16

Breakfast	Lunch	Dinner	Snacks	Drinks
2 eggs (scrambled, fried, boiled) with 2–3 rashers of bacon and ½ an avocado	Mini Salami Pizzas (see recipe) with a large side salad dressed with olive oil and cider vinegar	Pork Stroganoff (see recipe; keep some for tomorrow) with Cauliflower Rice (see recipe)	**Consume up to 2 snacks per day and only when hungry** 10 olives Up to 30g hard cheese 10 Parmesan Crisps with 1 tbsp homemade Guacamole or homemade salsa ½ an avocado topped with balsamic vinegar 50g nuts (not peanuts) 1 Fat Bomb	6–8 glasses of water Tea and coffee (herbal or decaf if you prefer) In coffee and tea, try sticking with double cream or unsweetened almond or coconut milk

DAY 17

Breakfast	Lunch	Dinner	Snacks	Drinks
2–3 eggs scrambled with 2 tbsp double cream, 1 handful of chives and spinach served with 50g salmon (optional)	Salad (salad leaves, cucumber, peppers, tomatoes, celery) with any protein option (around 100–150g) with lemon and olive oil dressing – can also sprinkle some seeds on top	Pork Stroganoff (left over from last night's dinner) with Cauliflower Rice	**Consume up to 2 snacks per day and only when hungry** 10 olives Up to 30g hard cheese 10 Parmesan Crisps with 1 tbsp homemade Guacamole or homemade salsa ½ an avocado topped with balsamic vinegar 50g nuts (not peanuts) 1 Fat Bomb	6–8 glasses of water Tea and coffee (herbal or decaf if you prefer) In coffee and tea, try sticking with double cream or unsweetened almond or coconut milk

Breakfast	Lunch	Dinner	Snacks	Drinks
Warm Chia Seed Breakfast Mug (see recipe)	Chorizo (up to 50g), red pepper and goats' cheese (30g) 2–3 egg omelette	Creamy Mushroom and Ham 'Pasta' (see recipe)	**Consume up to 2 snacks per day and only when hungry** 10 olives Up to 30g hard cheese 10 Parmesan Crisps with 1 tbsp homemade Guacamole or homemade salsa ½ an avocado topped with balsamic vinegar 50g nuts (not peanuts) 1 Fat Bomb	6–8 glasses of water Tea and coffee (herbal or decaf if you prefer) In coffee and tea, try sticking with double cream or unsweetened almond or coconut milk

Breakfast	Lunch	Dinner	Snacks	Drinks
Egg, salmon and avocado platter: 3 eggs (cooked any way you like), 50g salmon (any kind) ½ an avocado and 6 cherry tomatoes	Steak (100g uncooked weight) and blue cheese salad: (up to 30g cheese), 1 handful of young spinach leaves, 1 handful of rocket, ½ green pepper, 50g cucumber, 3 celery stalks	2 large flat mushrooms stuffed with mozzarella, topped with herbs of your choice and grilled, served with 2 portions of vegetables	**Consume up to 2 snacks per day and only when hungry** 10 olives Up to 30g hard cheese 10 Parmesan Crisps with 1 tbsp homemade Guacamole or homemade salsa ½ an avocado topped with balsamic vinegar 50g nuts (not peanuts) 1 Fat Bomb	6–8 glasses of water Tea and coffee (herbal or decaf if you prefer) In coffee and tea, try sticking with double cream or unsweetened almond or coconut milk

Breakfast	Lunch	Dinner	Snacks	Drinks
3 tbsp natural whole-milk yogurt with 50g sugar-free granola	Salad (salad leaves, cucumber, peppers, tomatoes, celery) with any protein option (around 100–150g) with lemon and olive oil dressing – can also sprinkle some seeds on top	Lamb Koftas (see recipe) served with a small Greek salad and 1 tbsp of crème fraîche	**Consume up to 2 snacks per day and only when hungry** 10 olives Up to 30g hard cheese 10 Parmesan Crisps with 1 tbsp homemade Guacamole or homemade salsa ½ an avocado topped with balsamic vinegar 50g nuts (not peanuts) 1 Fat Bomb	6–8 glasses of water Tea and coffee (herbal or decaf if you prefer) In coffee and tea, try sticking with double cream or unsweetened almond or coconut milk

Breakfast	Lunch	Dinner	Snacks	Drinks
Berry Smoothie (see recipe)	3 eggs scrambled with 2 handfuls of shredded spinach, 1 handful of chopped spring onions and 1 tbsp grated Parmesan, served with homemade salsa and a large salad	Chicken Parmesan served with 100g green beans and 100g mushrooms cooked in butter	**Consume up to 2 snacks per day and only when hungry** 10 olives Up to 30g hard cheese 10 Parmesan Crisps with 1 tbsp homemade Guacamole or homemade salsa ½ an avocado topped with balsamic vinegar 50g nuts (not peanuts) 1 Fat Bomb	6–8 glasses of water Tea and coffee (herbal or decaf if you prefer) In coffee and tea, try sticking with double cream or unsweetened almond or coconut milk

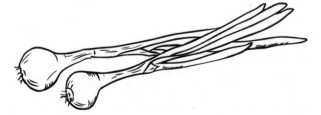

CHAPTER SEVEN

Breakfast	Lunch	Dinner	Snacks	Drinks
3 tbsp natural whole-milk (or Greek) yogurt mixed with 1 tbsp double cream (optional), 1 tbsp coconut flakes, 30g mixed nuts and 50g berries	Salad of rocket, spinach, black and green olives and up to 50g feta cheese with olive oil and vinegar dressing	Cheesy Courgette 'Pasta' (see recipe)	**Consume up to 2 snacks per day and only when hungry** 10 olives Up to 30g hard cheese ½ an avocado topped with balsamic vinegar 50g nuts (not peanuts) 1 Fat Bomb	6–8 glasses of water Tea and coffee (herbal or decaf if you prefer) In coffee and tea, try sticking with double cream or unsweetened almond or coconut milk

Breakfast	Lunch	Dinner	Snacks	Drinks
Warm Chia Seed Breakfast Mug (see recipe)	Green Smoothie (see recipe) with 3 celery stalks and almond butter	Shallow-Fried Coconut Camembert (see recipe) served with salad leaves	**Consume up to 2 snacks per day and only when hungry** 10 olives Up to 30g hard cheese ½ an avocado topped with balsamic vinegar 50g nuts (not peanuts) 1 Fat Bomb	6–8 glasses of water Tea and coffee (herbal or decaf if you prefer) In coffee and tea, try sticking with double cream or unsweetened almond or coconut milk

Breakfast	Lunch	Dinner	Snacks	Drinks
3 eggs scrambled with 3 chopped spring onions, 1 large handful of shredded spinach and some snipped chives	Beetroot and goat's cheese salad: 50g goat's cheese, 50g diced fresh beetroot, 30g walnuts, 2 large handfuls of young spinach leaves, 1 handful of rocket, ½ a green pepper, 50g cucumber, with olive oil and cider vinegar dressing (3 parts oil to 1 vinegar)	2 large mushrooms stuffed with mozzarella and ricotta cheese, and herbs of your choice, and grilled served with a large salad	**Consume up to 2 snacks per day and only when hungry** 10 olives Up to 30g hard cheese ½ an avocado topped with balsamic vinegar 50g nuts (not peanuts) 1 Fat Bomb	6–8 glasses of water Tea and coffee (herbal or decaf if you prefer) In coffee and tea, try sticking with double cream or unsweetened almond or coconut milk

Breakfast	Lunch	Dinner	Snacks	Drinks
3 tbsp natural whole-milk yogurt mixed with 1 tbsp almond butter, 1 tbsp coconut flakes, 30g mixed nuts and seeds and 50g berries	Green Smoothie (see recipe) with 3 celery stalks and almond butter	Baked Eggs with Asparagus and Mozzarella (see recipe)	**Consume up to 2 snacks per day and only when hungry** 10 olives Up to 30g hard cheese ½ an avocado topped with balsamic vinegar 50g nuts (not peanuts) 1 Fat Bomb	6–8 glasses of water Tea and coffee (herbal or decaf if you prefer) In coffee and tea, try sticking with double cream or unsweetened almond or coconut milk

Breakfast	Lunch	Dinner	Snacks	Drinks
Spiced omelette: 3 large eggs whisked with 4 tsp milk or double cream, finely chopped onion and red pepper, coriander, cumin and ½–1 tsp chilli powder. Serve with fresh salad or guacamole	Grilled halloumi salad: up to 60g halloumi with 2 large handfuls of young spinach leaves, 1 handful of rocket, ½ a green pepper, 50g cucumber, with olive oil and cider vinegar dressing (3 parts oil to 1 vinegar)	Aubergine 'pizzas': cut aubergine into 1cm discs (up to 8 slices), spread with sundried tomato paste, top with a slice of mozzarella and a slice of Cheddar cheese and sprinkle basil on top. Grill for 5–10 minutes. Serve with sautéed spinach	**Consume up to 2 snacks per day and only when hungry** 10 olives Up to 30g hard cheese ½ an avocado topped with balsamic vinegar 50g nuts (not peanuts) 1 Fat Bomb	6–8 glasses of water Tea and coffee (herbal or decaf if you prefer) In coffee and tea, try sticking with double cream or unsweetened almond or coconut milk

Breakfast	Lunch	Dinner	Snacks	Drinks
3 tbsp natural whole-milk (or Greek) yogurt mixed with 1 tbsp double cream (optional), 1 tbsp coconut flakes, 30g mixed nuts and 50g berries	Super Green Soup (see recipe)	Cauliflower Mushroom Risotto (see recipe) with Parmesan cheese	**Consume up to 2 snacks per day and only when hungry** 10 olives Up to 30g hard cheese ½ an avocado topped with balsamic vinegar 50g nuts (not peanuts) 1 Fat Bomb	6–8 glasses of water Tea and coffee (herbal or decaf if you prefer) In coffee and tea, try sticking with double cream or unsweetened almond or coconut milk

CHAPTER SEVEN

Breakfast	Lunch	Dinner	Snacks	Drinks
Berry Smoothie	Egg 'muffins': whisk together 4 eggs, chopped tomato, green pepper and onion. Pour into buttered muffin tins and fill halfway. Bake in the oven at 160°C for 15 minutes or until cooked	One red pepper stuffed with mushrooms and spinach creamed together with 50ml double cream and 1 tsp butter, baked with 50g mozzarella and 50g feta cheese for 10 minutes at 180°C	**Consume up to 2 snacks per day and only when hungry** 10 olives Up to 30g hard cheese ½ an avocado topped with balsamic vinegar 50g nuts (not peanuts) 1 Fat Bomb	6–8 glasses of water Tea and coffee (herbal or decaf if you prefer). In coffee and tea, try sticking with double cream or unsweetened almond or coconut milk

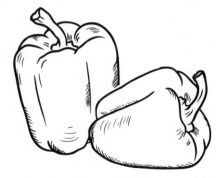

8   How do I manage my emotions?

The eight-
week plan
Week 4

Emotions are those scary things we don't like to talk about, sometimes not even to our closest friends and families. Particularly if those emotions are fear, shame and guilt. During this week we'll give you insights into your emotional habits as well as tools to help you change these habits.

Human emotions

We are human beings and it's natural to have a range of emotions, from happiness and joy to sadness and pessimism. Whatever your state of mind or general disposition this week, I want to help you stay in touch with these emotions. When you feel sad, depressed or full of grief or fear, it's important to sit with the emotion. You don't have to fix it straight away. It's OK to feel that way. As addicts we've learnt to suppress emotions when they're too overwhelming. We then act out our addiction by binge eating or consuming sugary foods or withholding food – we want to distract ourselves, deaden ourselves, as a solution to managing our emotions.

When you feel an emotion that's scary, don't immediately distract yourself with something. Just sit. This may feel really unnerving. Perhaps take out your journal and write down how you're feeling: did anything trigger it, where in your body do you feel the emotion? Reassure yourself that it's OK to feel this way; it's natural and normal. Importantly, there's nothing to fix. Be accepting and kind to yourself.

You may only be able to do this for a minute at first – but as you do it more you'll start to build up emotional muscles. Over time you'll feel less and less inclined to 'act out' when you experience an overwhelming emotion.

If you feel completely overwhelmed by your emotions, if you feel you're unable to live a fulfilling life because you are mired in negative emotions, please seek help – we've listed some resources at the beginning of this book.

We've only talked about 'negative' emotions but it's also important to acknowledge your positive emotions – joy, happiness, pride and exuberance. Sit with that emotion too – don't run away from it – let it fill up all corners of your life. You may even want to journal about it. Just remember you'll experience a wide range of emotions but they're not

Karen

I've always been emotionally reactive. When I feel attacked or criticised I immediately lash out verbally, although I often deeply regret what I say. Now when I feel criticised or upset by another person's words or behaviour I choose to take 'time out'. I remove myself from the situation and go for a walk, spend time in nature or listen to soothing music. I ask myself: Will this matter in a year's time? Most of the time it won't, so I then don't need to waste more time or energy on the situation. Instead of reacting I'm choosing to respond in a way that empowers rather than disempowers me. Sometimes I do need to confront the person about the way they have treated me and then I choose my words carefully. I state my feelings and then let it go. I love the saying: 'Say what you mean, mean what you say, but don't be mean when you say it'.

Journal exercise

Take a few minutes to reflect on your emotional reactions – how do you react when you're feeling overwhelmed or out of control? List those situations that are emotionally charged for you. For example, when your wife or husband comes home late from work, or when you're criticised. Which situations press your emotional buttons?

permanent. Treat your feelings as visitors, each one coming to teach you something. Welcome each and every one of them and know that they will leave once they are ready. Don't get attached to them – look at the lessons they're bringing.

We've all learnt emotional responses through the experiences in our lives. But they are only habits – and like other habits, we can learn to change them.

Emotional maturity

What are we trying to achieve with these emotions? As addicts we use emotions as a way of controlling ourselves, as an excuse to binge. Think about the last time you had a binge session. What was the triggering emotion: Anger? Fear? Loneliness? Guilt? Shame?

We also use emotions to control others. For example, anger is a great tool for manipulating others: if I get angry then people will be

scared and do what I want. We learnt this kind of behaviour as toddlers, before we knew how to regulate our emotions and ask for what we want.

As addicts we revert to child-like behaviours because we haven't learnt emotional maturity. We think it's OK to bully, to demand unrealistic things of other people, to be overly critical, to be passive-aggressive, egocentric, self-righteous or always be right. Did you recognise yourself in that list?

Managing your emotions

In any recovery process it's important to take responsibility for your emotions. I've put together a simple three-step model illustrated and explained on the next page to help you manage your emotions.

JOURNAL EXERCISE

Reflect on the following questions to get a better understanding of yourself and your emotional maturity:

1   What are you like at home? Are you generally caring and kind to your family? Or are you a bully? Do you sulk? Lose your temper often? Do you play the victim? Do you always expect things to go your way?
2   What are you like at work? Are you generally supportive and caring in your work environment? Are you enthusiastic and friendly? Overly demanding? Uptight? Secretive? Overly critical?
3   What are you like with friends or groups to which you belong? Do you try and rescue everyone?
4   What are you like with yourself? Are you manipulative? Or do you show genuine kindness and compassion towards yourself?
5   Are you ruled by whichever emotion is present or are you able to remove yourself from the situation and see the bigger picture?

I acknowledge how I am feeling > **I take responsibility** for my feelings (including my reactions to other people's emotions) > **I express** my emotions in a way that honours my needs and respects others (adult to adult)

Let's look at how you can apply these in a practical way:

SCENARIO ONE
Your husband or wife continually comes home from work late. Your reaction until now has been to pretend nothing is wrong, to phone and nag him or her to come home, or to shout and scream once they do.

What if you said this instead?
'When you come home late from work and don't let me know, I worry that something has

happened to you. If I keep phoning you to find out where you are I feel like a nagging wife or husband keeping tabs on you – and I don't like being that person. Can we agree that if you are going to be more than 30 minutes late you'll call me?'

SCENARIO TWO

Your husband, wife, friend or parent teases you about your appearance, weight or what you're wearing. When this happens, often you get angry and retaliate. Or you sulk and clam up.

What if you said this instead?

'When you tease me about my appearance and weight – whether in front of other people or in private – I feel you don't respect me or love me. I'm trying to make positive changes in my life and I really need your support to make this a success.'

SCENARIO THREE

You have a heated discussion or argument with someone and it blows up – you end up calling each other names. Perhaps it gets physical. Or you storm out of the room. You never come back to the disagreement – until the next time you have an argument.

What if you said this instead?

'Right now I'm too angry to have a rational conversation. Can we please agree on some time out right now, and talk again in an hour?'

JOURNAL EXERCISE

During one of the previous journal exercises in this chapter, you listed situations that are emotionally charged for you. Identify how you can address the situation in a positive way: what is the discussion you could have with the other person?

Situation: 'When this happens . . . '

Feelings: 'This is how I feel . . . '

Express needs: 'Can we agree . . . '

You don't have to address all these situations at once – pick a relatively easy one to address this week. Start building up your emotional muscle.

Deirdre's story

My entire life has been a struggle with weight gain and loss. As a little girl I was very upset when we did PE at school – my legs touched at the top where my friend had a big gap. I tried to stand with bandy legs so that the top of my thighs would have a gap. I always felt fat.

My parents both tried to help me keep my weight down. My mother hid chocolates and biscuits away from me, but when she went out I would climb on a chair and look for the hidden goodies. They once arranged for me to fly to see a doctor in Johannesburg who gave injections for weight loss. All this was done to help me. Diet pills, weight-loss groups, health farms – I always found a way to cheat. I was even hospitalised to lose weight. Yo-yo dieting and weight loss – this was my life. I felt disconnected from the glamorous and beautiful circle of people that my dad, Christiaan Barnard, moved in.

Journal exercise

What other positive activities can you identify to use to switch your attention?

My wonderful daughter, Karen Thomson, started the HELP Program with Professor Tim Noakes. She fed me information, we attended lectures by Professor Noakes and she sent me excellent articles to read. The entire programme just made sense to me. I increased my fat intake, which actually took away cravings and my continuous hunger. Magic! I have not been well, but I feel much better on the LCHF way of eating.

When I have relapsed and eaten something sugary, I've had an immense desire and craving for more. I find I don't crave carbs. But sugar, yes. I am also addicted to chocolate. I can't take just one piece. I must finish the chocolate, whether it is a large or small bar. I no longer keep any temptation in my home.

I have lost 10kg, but more importantly I feel much better. I am at peace with who I am and for the first time in my life I have hope and confidence that the yo-yo weight will be gone. I don't get hungry and if I relapse I can get myself back on track without anxiety.

★

Tips for managing overheated emotions

In this chapter I've talked about the importance of recognising and honouring your emotions, about staying connected to them. But sometimes when emotions get overheated it's useful to switch your attention to something else to bring down the heat. Our tendency is to reach for our favourite food – but what else can we do?

- Watch your favourite film
- Listen to loud music
- Move: walk, dance, swim, run, twirl around your lounge, climb up and down the stairs a few times
- Punch or scream into a cushion.

WEEKLY JOURNAL EXERCISE

Take a few minutes to reflect on your week and this stage of your journey:

1   What were your greatest successes this week?
2   How will you build on your successes?
3   Did you stick to your meal plan?
4   Did you maintain abstinence from sugar and carbs?
5   If not, what triggered you to relapse or slip?
    What have you learnt from this experience?
6   What exercise did you do this week?
7   Are you unhappy about anything that happened this week?
8   Have you been affirming yourself?
9   What will you do differently next week to support your journey in recovery positively?
10 Make a list of ten things you are grateful for.

♥

Affirmation
I am grateful for all my emotions and learn from each and every one.

USEFUL RESOURCES

Quit Comfort Eating: Lose Weight By Managing Your Emotions by Dr Susan Albers (Piatkus, 2013). Low emotional intelligence can lock you into a vicious cycle of dieting failure. In this book Dr Albers explores how to combat the most common emotional barriers to weight loss.

Dark Nights of the Soul: A Guide to Finding Your Way Through Life's Ordeals by Thomas Moore (Piatkus, 2004). This book offers valuable advice on how to use trying times as an opportunity to reflect and delve into the soul's deepest needs. And ultimately, to find new understanding and meaning.

DAY 22

Breakfast	Lunch	Dinner	Snacks	Drinks
Warm Chia Seed Breakfast Mug (see recipe)	Salad (salad leaves, cucumber, peppers, tomatoes, celery) with any protein option (100–150g) with lemon and olive oil dressing – can also sprinkle some seeds on top	2 eggs scrambled with 50g salmon, 50g shredded spinach, 4 florets of broccoli and 25g butter	**Consume up to 2 snacks per day and only when hungry** 10 olives Up to 30g hard cheese 10 Parmesan Crisps with 1 tbsp homemade Guacamole or homemade salsa ½ an avocado topped with balsamic vinegar 50g nuts (not peanuts) 1 Fat Bomb	6–8 glasses of water Tea and coffee (herbal or decaf if you prefer) In coffee and tea, try sticking with double cream or unsweetened almond or coconut milk

DAY 23

Breakfast	Lunch	Dinner	Snacks	Drinks
2 Egg and Parma Ham Cups (see recipe) served with 1 handful of spinach wilted with 2 tsp butter	Super Green Soup (see recipe) with 1 slice Nut and Seed Loaf (see recipe)	Smoked salmon and cream cheese stir-fry: stir-fry ½ a red pepper. ½ a green pepper, ½ a yellow pepper, asparagus, kale and red onion; stir in 75g smoked salmon and 30g cream cheese and season to taste; top with grated Parmesan cheese (optional)	**Consume up to 2 snacks per day and only when hungry** 10 olives Up to 30g hard cheese 10 Parmesan Crisps with 1 tbsp homemade Guacamole or homemade salsa ½ an avocado topped with balsamic vinegar 50g nuts (not peanuts) 1 Fat Bomb	6–8 glasses of water Tea and coffee (herbal or decaf if you prefer) In coffee and tea, try sticking with double cream or unsweetened almond or coconut milk

DAY 24

Breakfast	Lunch	Dinner	Snacks	Drinks
3 tbsp natural whole-milk yogurt with 50g sugar-free Nut Granola (see recipe) and 50g berries	Creamy Avocado Soup with 2 Seed Crackers (see recipes)	Chicken 'fajitas': stir-fry chicken strips (plain) with sliced red onion (¼) and red pepper (½), seasoned with salt, cumin and paprika. Serve in iceberg lettuce leaves, topped with guacamole (1 tbsp) and salsa (1 tbsp)	**Consume up to 2 snacks per day and only when hungry** 10 olives Up to 30g hard cheese 10 Parmesan Crisps with 1 tbsp homemade Guacamole or homemade salsa ½ an avocado topped with balsamic vinegar 50g nuts (not peanuts) 1 Fat Bomb	6–8 glasses of water Tea and coffee (herbal or decaf if you prefer) In coffee and tea, try sticking with double cream or unsweetened almond or coconut milk

Breakfast	Lunch	Dinner	Snacks	Drinks
3 rashers of bacon with 50g cream cheese and 50g berries	1 Mocha Protein (see recipe) or Green Smoothie (see recipe)	Tomato and Prawn 'Pasta' (see recipe)	**Consume up to 2 snacks per day and only when hungry** 10 olives Up to 30g hard cheese 10 Parmesan Crisps with 1 tbsp homemade Guacamole or homemade salsa ½ an avocado topped with balsamic vinegar 50g nuts (not peanuts) 1 Fat Bomb	6–8 glasses of water Tea and coffee (herbal or decaf if you prefer) In coffee and tea, try sticking with double cream or unsweetened almond or coconut milk

Breakfast	Lunch	Dinner	Snacks	Drinks
Egg, salmon and avocado platter: 3 eggs (cooked any way you like), 50g salmon (any kind), ½ an avocado and 6 cherry tomatoes	Steak (100g uncooked weight) and blue cheese salad: (up to 30g cheese), 1 handful of young spinach leaves, 1 handful of rocket, ½ a green pepper, 50g cucumber, 3 celery stalks	Crème Fraîche and Coriander Chicken (see recipe) served with a large side salad drizzled with 1 tbsp of olive oil	**Consume up to 2 snacks per day and only when hungry** 10 olives Up to 30g hard cheese 10 Parmesan Crisps with 1 tbsp homemade Guacamole or homemade salsa ½ an avocado topped with balsamic vinegar 50g nuts (not peanuts) 1 Fat Bomb	6–8 glasses of water Tea and coffee (herbal or decaf if you prefer) In coffee and tea, try sticking with double cream or unsweetened almond or coconut milk

Breakfast	Lunch	Dinner	Snacks	Drinks
3 tbsp natural whole-milk yogurt with 50g sugar-free granola with 50g berries	Warm goat's cheese and walnut salad: 30g goat's cheese, 30g walnuts, 1 handful of young spinach leaves, 1 handful of rocket, ½ a green pepper, 50g cucumber, 3 celery stalks	Spanish omelette: 3 eggs mixed with diced 30g chorizo, chopped red pepper (½) and paprika; served topped with cream cheese (30g)	**Consume up to 2 snacks per day and only when hungry** 10 olives Up to 30g hard cheese 10 Parmesan Crisps with 1 tbsp homemade Guacamole or homemade salsa ½ an avocado topped with balsamic vinegar 50g nuts (not peanuts) 1 Fat Bomb	6–8 glasses of water Tea and coffee (herbal or decaf if you prefer) In coffee and tea, try sticking with double cream or unsweetened almond or coconut milk

Breakfast	Lunch	Dinner	Snacks	Drinks
3 eggs scrambled with butter, mixed with ½ an avocado, chopped ½ red pepper and 30g feta cheese	Thai Green Curry (see recipe) with 1–2 seed crackers or 1 slice of Nut and Seed Loaf (see recipe)	Portuguese style Piri-Piri Chicken (see recipe) with Cauliflower Rice (see recipe), pancetta, Brussels sprouts and garlic	**Consume up to 2 snacks per day and only when hungry** 10 olives Up to 30g hard cheese 10 Parmesan Crisps with 1 tbsp homemade Guacamole or homemade salsa ½ an avocado topped with balsamic vinegar 50g nuts (not peanuts) 1 Fat Bomb	6–8 glasses of water Tea and coffee (herbal or decaf if you prefer) In coffee and tea, try sticking with double cream or unsweetened almond or coconut milk

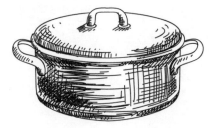

CHAPTER EIGHT

DAY 22

Breakfast	Lunch	Dinner	Snacks	Drinks
3 tbsp natural whole-milk (or Greek) yogurt mixed with 50g sugar-free Nut Granola (see recipe) and 50g of berries	Mediterranean vegetables (peppers, aubergine, onions and courgettes) and halloumi skewers served with a large salad dressed with olive oil and balsamic vinegar	2 Spinach and Courgette Burgers (see recipe) topped with Cheddar cheese and served with a large salad drizzled with olive oil	**Consume up to 2 snacks per day and only when hungry** 10 olives Up to 30g hard cheese ½ an avocado topped with balsamic vinegar 50g nuts (not peanuts) 1 Fat Bomb	6–8 glasses of water Tea and coffee (herbal or decaf if you prefer) In coffee and tea, try sticking with double cream or unsweetened almond or coconut milk

DAY 23

Breakfast	Lunch	Dinner	Snacks	Drinks
Egg 'muffins': whisk together 4 eggs, chopped tomato, green pepper and onion. Pour into buttered muffin tins and fill halfway. Bake in the oven at 160°C for 15 minutes or until cooked	Creamy Avocado Soup (see recipe) with 2 slices of Nut and Seed loaf (see recipe)	2 slices of Vegetarian Pizza (see recipe), served with Celeriac Chips (see recipe)	**Consume up to 2 snacks per day and only when hungry** 10 olives Up to 30g hard cheese ½ an avocado topped with balsamic vinegar 50g nuts (not peanuts) 1 Fat Bomb	6–8 glasses of water Tea and coffee (herbal or decaf if you prefer) In coffee and tea, try sticking with double cream or unsweetened almond or coconut milk

DAY 24

Breakfast	Lunch	Dinner	Snacks	Drinks
3 tbsp natural whole-milk (or Greek) yogurt mixed with 1 tbsp double cream (optional), 1 tbsp coconut flakes, 30g mixed nuts and 50g berries	Spring onion scrambled eggs: up to 3 eggs scrambled with coconut milk, mixed with chopped spring onion and sprinkled with fresh dill	Cream cheese and vegetable stir-fry: Stir-fry together 1 handful of spinach, 1 handful of kale, ½ a courgette, ½ a red pepper, ½ a yellow pepper, ½ a green pepper, 2 cloves of garlic and ¼ of an onion. Stir in 50g cream cheese and 50g mozzarella cheese and top with 30g walnuts and sunflower seeds	**Consume up to 2 snacks per day and only when hungry** 10 olives Up to 30g hard cheese ½ an avocado topped with balsamic vinegar 50g nuts (not peanuts) 1 Fat Bomb	6–8 glasses of water Tea and coffee (herbal or decaf if you prefer) In coffee and tea, try sticking with double cream or unsweetened almond or coconut milk

Breakfast	Lunch	Dinner	Snacks	Drinks
Warm Chia Seed Breakfast Mug (see recipe)	Green Smoothie (see recipe) with 3 celery stalks and almond butter	Spiced omelette: 3 large eggs whisked with 4 tsp milk or double cream, finely chopped onion and red pepper, coriander, cumin and ½–1 tsp chilli powder. Serve with homemade salsa or guacamole	**Consume up to 2 snacks per day and only when hungry** 10 olives Up to 30g hard cheese ½ an avocado topped with balsamic vinegar 50g nuts (not peanuts) 1 fat bomb	6–8 glasses of water Tea and coffee (herbal or decaf if you prefer) In coffee and tea, try sticking with double cream or unsweetened almond or coconut milk

Breakfast	Lunch	Dinner	Snacks	Drinks
Berry Smoothie (see recipe)	Super Green Soup (see recipe) served with 1 slice of Nut and Seed Loaf (see recipe) with butter	Aubergine 'pizzas': cut aubergine into 1cm discs (up to 8 slices), spread with sun-dried tomato paste, top with a slice of mozzarella and a slice of Cheddar cheese and sprinkle with basil. Grill for 5–10 minutes. Serve with sautéed spinach	**Consume up to 2 snacks per day and only when hungry** 10 olives Up to 30g hard cheese ½ an avocado topped with balsamic vinegar 50g nuts (not peanuts) 1 fat bomb	6–8 glasses of water Tea and coffee (herbal or decaf if you prefer) In coffee and tea, try sticking with double cream or unsweetened almond or coconut milk

Breakfast	Lunch	Dinner	Snacks	Drinks
Egg and avocado platter: 3 eggs (cooked any way you like) and ½ an avocado, and 6 cherry tomatoes	Caprese Salad (see recipe)	Mushroom Stroganoff (see recipe) with Cauliflower Rice (see recipe)	**Consume up to 2 snacks per day and only when hungry** 10 olives Up to 30g hard cheese ½ an avocado topped with balsamic vinegar 50g nuts (not peanuts) 1 fat bomb	6–8 glasses of water Tea and coffee (herbal or decaf if you prefer) In coffee and tea, try sticking with double cream or unsweetened almond or coconut milk

Breakfast	Lunch	Dinner	Snacks	Drinks
3 tbsp natural whole-milk (or Greek) yogurt mixed with 1 tbsp double cream (optional), 1 tbsp coconut flakes, 30g mixed nuts and 50g berries	Sugar-free Bruschetta (see recipe)	Sweet Potato Frittata (see recipe)	**Consume up to 2 snacks per day and only when hungry** 10 olives Up to 30g hard cheese ½ an avocado topped with balsamic vinegar 50g nuts (not peanuts) 1 fat bomb	6–8 glasses of water Tea and coffee (herbal or decaf if you prefer) In coffee and tea, try sticking with double cream or unsweetened almond or coconut milk

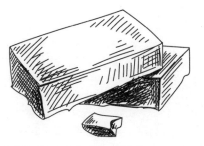

9   Love myself

When you've been in active addiction for a long time the last thing you can think about is loving yourself. During Week Five I'll provide simple ways to help boost your self-esteem and guide you towards a little bit more self-loving.

What is self-esteem?

I like to define self-esteem as a positive belief in myself, something that gives me confidence and enables me to be inwardly caring and supportive. It's also a belief that I'm worthy of recovery, of being in a loving relationship (with myself and others) and of happiness and joy.

Negative self-esteem can hinder us in so many ways: it hampers our persistence to push through the difficult times in recovery because we don't 'deserve' it; it encourages staying in abusive or negative relationships because we lack the ability to see ourselves in a loving relationship; we don't try to get promotions because we haven't got the 'skills' despite being an excellent candidate; or we become doormats for people because we can't stand up for ourselves.

When we're in active addiction we often have a very negative self-esteem. Over the next few pages we'll look at the link between trauma and addiction and how that impacts on your self-esteem. We'll also examine how you can start changing your self-belief.

Trauma and addiction

Recent studies have shown that addiction and trauma, specifically childhood trauma, are strongly linked. The term may seem alarming but let's look at some trauma examples:

- Being bullied at school: emotionally, physically or psychologically
- Being rejected by friends
- Your parents forgetting to fetch you from a party or play date
- Experiencing violence such as a hijacking or robbery
- A family member or friend leaving
- Surgery
- Death
- Being in a accident (even if small or you didn't sustain major injuries)

Most of us have experienced trauma to some extent. Trauma is also subjective: what one person experiences as traumatic may not feel the same for someone else. The common thread joining trauma and addiction is that trauma instils a sense of fear. It's often deep-rooted and results in pain and suffering. So we dissociate by mentally and physically disconnecting from our identities and ourselves. As food addicts desperately attempting to cope with this fear and angst, we start using self-destructive habits such as overeating, comfort eating and binge eating.

Through these traumatic and fear-creating experiences we start to believe there is something intrinsically wrong with us, that we are not lovable, acceptable or worthwhile. We're left with an unbalanced perspective of ourselves. We stop believing in our ability to make sound decisions. We stop living full, meaningful lives. These are negative core beliefs, things that motivate us to behave, think and feel in addictive ways.

Know that you are good enough

Negative core beliefs are different for each person, but generally they make you believe that who you are isn't good enough. Consider these examples:

- I'm not OK the way I am
- I'm not lovable
- I'm not good enough
- My feelings aren't important
- I need something outside of me to feel happy and complete

Karen

I came into recovery with a shattered sense of self and no self-esteem. I operated from the core belief 'I am worthless'. My behaviours, thoughts and feelings all supported this belief. I abused myself and landed up in relationships where that belief was reinforced.

When I entered rehab, my counsellor helped me identify my fear-based belief system and formulated a specific affirmation to help me to start believing in myself. Every day before breakfast, lunch and dinner I had to look at myself in front of a mirror and repeat the following sentence five times: 'My name is Karen, I am a good person. I don't need to please others. God [call on any greater power you believe in], teach me to love myself.'

I cannot adequately explain just how hard it was to look myself in the eye and acknowledge the pain and suffering I had caused myself. The process was tough but something in me shifted and my core belief started changing. I started operating (thinking, feeling and believing) from a place of love for myself, and in turn was able to start treating others with love and respect. Addiction robbed me of my self-worth and self-esteem; recovery enabled me to restore it.

By buying into negative core beliefs – and consequently addictive thought systems – we see ourselves as lacking or incomplete. We don't feel we can deal with our own emotions. This begins an external search to fill the gaps and we start 'self-medicating' with sugar and carbohydrates (or other substances). Our addictions are born out of thinking we are less than whole.

Babies aren't born hating themselves. As addicts, how do we find a way back to being in love with ourselves, so that even our own fingers and toes can seem delightful and a source of wonder? It's an ongoing process, but you'll experience the greatest freedom once you realise that achieving freedom internally is the only solution. No food, person or drug will be able to give you high self-esteem; it's up to you. Happiness is an inside job.

Gradually realising that you're a beautiful, capable and worth-while person is one of the greatest gifts you will give yourself and those around you. Moving from a base of fear to a base of love creates amazing opportunities to open up in every area of your life. By going within to discover and restore ourselves to a natural way of being, we give ourselves permission to be the very best we can be in whichever roles we choose for ourselves. It also opens the way for people around us to behave in positive and authentic ways.

Self-love, self-worth and self-acceptance can only come from the *self*. It requires dedication and practice.

★

Tips for when you're invited out to eat
There are few situations more awkward than being invited to someone's home for dinner and not being able to eat any of the food they have graciously prepared. To avoid embarrassment to both parties it's important to plan ahead.

You may have shared the letter you created during Week One with close friends and family. But what do you do when your hosts are unaware of your lifestyle change? My suggestion is simple: phone or email them and politely ask what they're preparing for dinner and whether you can bring anything – suggest a delicious salad or sugar-free dessert. If you feel the need to explain why you're asking, then do so. Keep your explanation short and simple. 'I've changed my eating habits and no longer eat sugar and carbs, but I'm more than happy to bring a dish.' Remember, it's more important to hold yourself and your health in high esteem than to please others.

JOURNAL EXERCISE

- Can you identify a core belief that you operate from? Take time to think of one that really resonates with you. This is a thought or feeling that has likely been with you for most of your life. It's not positive and is often deeply ingrained.
- Write down your core belief.
- You've probably been behaving, thinking and feeling according to this belief for most of your life. Can you accept how damaging this must have been for you?
- Are you ready to let go of this negative core belief and replace it with a positive, empowering core belief?
- Look at your negative core belief and formulate an empowering, positive belief to oppose it. For example, if your core belief is 'I'm not good enough' then your positive statement could be 'I am good enough exactly as I am'. If your core belief is 'my feelings are not important' then your positive response could be '*all* my feelings are authentic and important.'
- Write your statement on sticky notes and post them in as many places as possible. On the bathroom mirror, your fridge, your car's rear view mirror . . . anywhere you'll be reminded of your new core belief. Say it often.

Here are more examples of positive core beliefs:

- I'm worthwhile
- I'm lovable
- I deserve to be treated with respect
- I accept myself as I am
- I have a right to express my feelings and emotions appropriately
- I am enough
- I love myself exactly as I am

Tania's story

My mother put me on my first diet when I was nine years old. I weighed 45kg and my goal weight was 39kg. Those six kilos took for ever to lose, but eventually, after months and months of attending weight-loss groups and meetings, I was at my goal weight.

That December we went away for the holidays. I remember eating every available sweet, chocolate and ice cream over that three-week holiday – it didn't take long for me to regain those hard-lost kilos. During the rest of my primary school years I embarked on a number of weight-loss systems: a concoction of tables, injections, groups, controlled programmes . . . There was nothing I could stick to.

I reached an absolute low point in 2013. My brother had broken his foot and I went to visit him, taking all his favourite treats. I remember standing over the kitchen counter just stuffing my mouth with all the sweets, biscuits and crisps I could manage. I wasn't hungry, but I could not control myself and had to finish everything.

The next day I googled food addictions and came across Karen Thomson and the HELP Program. I sent an email and Karen replied immediately saying they had a six-week session starting that afternoon. I'm not a spontaneous person and like everything planned. It was difficult for me to just drop everything and go, but it was the start of me locating the happier woman trapped inside for so many years.

It's been difficult to abstain from carbs and sugar, but it does get easier over time. I've learnt that the craving will pass and that the person I was while I was 'using' is not the woman I want to be. For me abstinence is not consuming sugar or carbohydrates. Abstinence is not overeating, or eating when I'm not hungry, or eating until I'm overly full.

My first relapse happened a few weeks into my recovery. I was making breakfast for a large group. I flipped some hash browns and unconsciously licked the spatula. There was no going back. I scoffed about six hash browns without taking a breath. Moments later my boyfriend came in and I yelled at him to please leave. The carbs had made me crazy and turned me into a monster. I'd wanted my 'fix' so scoffed all the hash browns I could lay my hands on. That was a crucial moment – I realised I cannot have 'just one' when it comes to carbs. It's all or nothing for me.

→

The HELP Program has helped me to realise my full potential. I no longer avoid social occasions and I've learnt to accept that being just me is OK: I am glorious and beautiful and I love myself, and my opinion is the only one that matters.

I'm learning to love every second of life and the beautiful blessings that each day brings. In my first year of recovery I completed my first triathlon and ran my first half-marathon. The old me wouldn't have dared to attempt such things. It doesn't matter what I weigh, this is who I want to be. The weight loss will come. Meanwhile, it's not going to stop me from living my life.

♥

Affirmation
I am confident and capable of making decisions that empower me.

WEEKLY JOURNAL EXERCISE

Take a few minutes to reflect on your week and this stage of your journey:

1. What were your greatest successes this week?
2. How will you build on your successes?
3. Did you stick to your meal plan?
4. Did you maintain abstinence from sugar and carbs?
5. If not, what triggered you to relapse or slip? What have you learnt from this experience?
6. What exercise did you do this week?
7. Are you unhappy about anything that happened this week?
8. Have you been affirming yourself?
9. What will you do differently next week to support your journey in recovery positively?
10. Make a list of ten things you are grateful for.

USEFUL RESOURCES

Courage: Overcoming Fear and Igniting Self-Confidence by Debbie Ford (HarperCollins, 2012). Written by a recovering addict with a deep understanding of addiction and low self-esteem, this book explores conquering fears, accepting flaws, and tapping into our true potential.

How to be an Adult: A Handbook for Psychological and Spiritual Integration by David Richo (Paulist Press, 1991). Full of psychological insights and spiritual wisdom, this book explores techniques that can be helpful in achieving psychological and spiritual health and wholeness.

DAY 29

Breakfast	Lunch	Dinner	Snacks	Drinks
3 tbsp natural whole-milk (or Greek) yogurt mixed with 1 tbsp double cream (optional), 1 tbsp coconut flakes, 30g mixed nuts and 50g berries	Tuna Niçoise Salad (see recipe)	Coconut chicken with mango, chilli salsa, served with a large green salad	**Consume up to 2 snacks per day and only when hungry** 10 olives Up to 30g hard cheese 10 Parmesan Crisps with 1 tbsp homemade Guacamole or homemade salsa ½ an avocado topped with balsamic vinegar 50g nuts (not peanuts) 1 Fat Bomb	6–8 glasses of water Tea and coffee (herbal or decaf if you prefer) In coffee and tea, try sticking with double cream or unsweetened almond or coconut milk

DAY 30

Breakfast	Lunch	Dinner	Snacks	Drinks
Egg, salmon and avocado platter: 3 eggs (cooked any way you like), 50g salmon (any kind), ½ an avocado and 6 cherry tomatoes	Chicken Tikka Strips (see recipe) served on a large bed of spinach, 50g cucumber and 8 cherry tomatoes with 1 tbsp crème fraîche on top	1 small steak (about 100g) served with a creamy mushroom sauce served with one handful of green beans cooked in 2tsp of butter	**Consume up to 2 snacks per day and only when hungry** 10 olives Up to 30g hard cheese 10 Parmesan Crisps with 1 tbsp homemade Guacamole or homemade salsa ½ an avocado topped with balsamic vinegar 50g nuts (not peanuts) 1 Fat Bomb	6–8 glasses of water Tea and coffee (herbal or decaf if you prefer) In coffee and tea, try sticking with double cream or unsweetened almond or coconut milk

DAY 31

Breakfast	Lunch	Dinner	Snacks	Drinks
Sugar-free Nut Granola (see recipe) (50g) with either unsweetened almond milk or 3tbsp of Greek yogurt with 50g of berries	Up to 5 Salmon Wraps: smoked salmon strips (up to 75g) spread with 2tsp of full-fat cream cheese and cucumber slices, rolled up	Chicken stuffed with ham and cheese served with roasted Mediterranean vegetables (aubergine, courgettes, peppers, red onion and tomatoes)	**Consume up to 2 snacks per day and only when hungry** 10 olives Up to 30g hard cheese 10 Parmesan Crisps with 1 tbsp homemade Guacamole or homemade salsa ½ an avocado topped with balsamic vinegar 50g nuts (not peanuts) 1 Fat Bomb	6–8 glasses of water Tea and coffee (herbal or decaf if you prefer) In coffee and tea, try sticking with double cream or unsweetened almond or coconut milk

Breakfast	Lunch	Dinner	Snacks	Drinks
3 rashers of bacon with 50g cream cheese and 50g blackberries	Sugar-free Bruschetta (see recipe)	Stuffed Goat's Cheese Turkey Burgers (see recipe) served with at least 2 portions of vegetables or a large salad	**Consume up to 2 snacks per day and only when hungry** 10 olives Up to 30g hard cheese 10 Parmesan Crisps with 1 tbsp homemade Guacamole or homemade salsa ½ an avocado topped with balsamic vinegar 50g nuts (not peanuts) 1 Fat Bomb	6–8 glasses of water Tea and coffee (herbal or decaf if you prefer) In coffee and tea, try sticking with double cream or unsweetened almond or coconut milk

Breakfast	Lunch	Dinner	Snacks	Drinks
2 eggs (cooked any way you like), 3 rashers of bacon, 1 good-quality sausage (at least 80% meat), 1 flat mushroom	Large prawn salad: up to 100g prawns with 3 handfuls of salad leaves, 50g cucumber and 8 cherry tomatoes with 2tbsp of olive oil and cider vinegar dressing	Creamy Mushroom and Ham 'Pasta' (see recipe)	**Consume up to 2 snacks per day and only when hungry** 10 olives Up to 30g hard cheese 10 Parmesan Crisps with 1 tbsp homemade Guacamole or homemade salsa ½ an avocado topped with balsamic vinegar 50g nuts (not peanuts) 1 Fat Bomb	6–8 glasses of water Tea and coffee (herbal or decaf if you prefer) In coffee and tea, try sticking with double cream or unsweetened almond or coconut milk

Breakfast	Lunch	Dinner	Snacks	Drinks
Egg, salmon and avocado platter: 3 eggs (cooked any way you like), 50g salmon (any kind) and ½ an avocado	Greek salad: half a cucumber, 10 cherry tomatoes halved, 50g feta cheese with 2–3tbsp of olive oil	Chicken breast stuffed with mozzarella (no more than 50g) wrapped in a slice of Parma ham or bacon then roasted for 20 mins at 180°C, served with 100g steamed green beans and 100g mushrooms cooked in butter	**Consume up to 2 snacks per day and only when hungry** 10 olives Up to 30g hard cheese 10 Parmesan Crisps with 1 tbsp homemade Guacamole or homemade salsa ½ an avocado topped with balsamic vinegar 50g nuts (not peanuts) 1 Fat Bomb	6–8 glasses of water Tea and coffee (herbal or decaf if you prefer) In coffee and tea, try sticking with double cream or unsweetened almond or coconut milk

Breakfast	Lunch	Dinner	Snacks	Drinks
Warm Chia Seed Breakfast Mug (see recipe) topped with 50g of berries (optional)	Grilled halloumi salad: up to 60g halloumi cheese with 2 large handfuls of young spinach leaves, 1 handful of rocket, ½ a green pepper, 50g cucumber, with olive oil and cider vinegar dressing (3 parts oil to 1 vinegar)	Spiced omelette: 3 large eggs whisked with 4 tsp or double cream, finely chopped onion and red pepper, coriander, cumin and ½–1 tsp chilli powder. Serve with fresh salad or guacamole	**Consume up to 2 snacks per day and only when hungry** 10 olives Up to 30g hard cheese 10 Parmesan Crisps with 1 tbsp homemade Guacamole or homemade salsa ½ an avocado topped with balsamic vinegar 50g nuts (not peanuts) 1 Fat Bomb	6–8 glasses of water Tea and coffee (herbal or decaf if you prefer) In coffee and tea, try sticking with double cream or unsweetened almond or coconut milk

Vegetarian Meal Plan Week 1 and 5

Breakfast	Lunch	Dinner	Snacks	Drinks
3 tbsp natural whole-milk (or Greek) yogurt mixed with 1 tbsp double cream (optional), 1 tbsp coconut flakes, 30g mixed nuts and 50g berries	Green Smoothie (see recipe) with 3 celery stalks and almond butter	Coconut Camembert with Berry Salad (see recipe)	**Consume up to 2 snacks per day and only when hungry** 10 olives Up to 30g hard cheese ½ an avocado topped with balsamic vinegar 50g nuts (not peanuts) 1 Fat Bomb	6–8 glasses of water Tea and coffee (herbal or decaf if you prefer) In coffee and tea, try sticking with double cream or unsweetened almond or coconut milk

Breakfast	Lunch	Dinner	Snacks	Drinks
1 egg 'muffin' (see recipe on p99 and add 150g chopped mushrooms that have been fried for 5 mins in butter)	Grilled halloumi salad: 60g halloumi, 2 large handfuls of young spinach leaves, 1 handful of rocket, ½ a green pepper, 50g cucumber, with olive oil and cider vinegar dressing (3 parts oil to 1 vinegar)	Aubergine 'pizzas': cut aubergine into 1cm discs (up to 8 slices), spread with sun-dried tomato paste, top with a slice of mozzarella and a slice of Cheddar cheese and sprinkle with basil. Grill for 5–10 minutes. Serve with sautéed spinach	**Consume up to 2 snacks per day and only when hungry** 10 olives Up to 30g hard cheese ½ an avocado topped with balsamic vinegar 50g nuts (not peanuts) 1 Fat Bomb	6–8 glasses of water Tea and coffee (herbal or decaf if you prefer) In coffee and tea, try sticking with double cream or unsweetened almond or coconut milk

Breakfast	Lunch	Dinner	Snacks	Drinks
3 tbsp natural whole-milk (or Greek) yogurt mixed with 1 tbsp double cream (optional), 1 tbsp coconut flakes, 30g mixed nuts and 50g berries	Beetroot and goat's cheese salad: 50g goat's cheese, 50g diced fresh beetroot, 30g walnuts, 2 large handfuls of young spinach leaves, 1 handful of rocket, ½ a green pepper, 50g cucumber, with olive oil and cider vinegar dressing (3 parts oil to 1 vinegar)	Baked eggs with asparagus and mozzarella (see recipe)	**Consume up to 2 snacks per day and only when hungry** 10 olives Up to 30g hard cheese ½ an avocado topped with balsamic vinegar 50g nuts (not peanuts) 1 Fat Bomb	6–8 glasses of water Tea and coffee (herbal or decaf if you prefer) In coffee and tea, try sticking with double cream or unsweetened almond or coconut milk

Breakfast	Lunch	Dinner	Snacks	Drinks
Warm Chia Seed Breakfast Mug (see recipe)	Cherry tomatoes (up to 10) stuffed with soft goat's cheese served with a large salad drizzled with olive oil and cider vinegar	Stuffed aubergine served on a large bed of spinach	**Consume up to 2 snacks per day and only when hungry** 10 olives Up to 30g hard cheese ½ an avocado topped with balsamic vinegar 50g nuts (not peanuts) 1 Fat Bomb	6–8 glasses of water Tea and coffee (herbal or decaf if you prefer) In coffee and tea, try sticking with double cream or unsweetened almond or coconut milk

Breakfast	Lunch	Dinner	Snacks	Drinks
3 tbsp natural whole-milk (or Greek) yogurt mixed with 1 tbsp double cream (optional), 1 tbsp coconut flakes, 30g mixed nuts and 50g berries	Warm goat's cheese salad: up to 60g goat's cheese, grilled and served with 2 large handfuls of young spinach leaves, 1 handful of rocket, ½ a green pepper, 50g cucumber, with olive oil and cider vinegar dressing (3 parts oil to 1 vinegar)	Chargrilled Mediterranean vegetables (aubergine, courgettes, peppers, red onion and tomatoes) and grilled halloumi served on a large bed of spinach sprinkled with walnuts and pumpkin seeds, with olive oil and cider vinegar dressing	**Consume up to 2 snacks per day and only when hungry** 10 olives Up to 30g hard cheese ½ an avocado topped with balsamic vinegar 50g nuts (not peanuts) 1 Fat Bomb	6–8 glasses of water Tea and coffee (herbal or decaf if you prefer) In coffee and tea, try sticking with double cream or unsweetened almond or coconut milk

Breakfast	Lunch	Dinner	Snacks	Drinks
Egg and avocado platter: 3 eggs (cooked any way you like), ½ an avocado and 6 cherry tomatoes	Green Smoothie (see recipe)	2 large flat mushrooms stuffed with mozzarella and ricotta cheese and herbs of your choice, and grilled. Served with a large salad	**Consume up to 2 snacks per day and only when hungry** 10 olives Up to 30g hard cheese ½ an avocado topped with balsamic vinegar 50g nuts (not peanuts) 1 Fat Bomb	6–8 glasses of water Tea and coffee (herbal or decaf if you prefer) In coffee and tea, try sticking with double cream or unsweetened almond or coconut milk

Breakfast	Lunch	Dinner	Snacks	Drinks
2 tbsp natural whole-milk (or Greek) yogurt mixed with 1 tbsp double cream (optional), 1 tbsp coconut flakes, 30g mixed nuts and 50g berries	Green Smoothie (see recipe)	Cheesy Courgette 'Pasta' (see recipe)	**Consume up to 2 snacks per day and only when hungry** 10 olives Up to 30g hard cheese ½ an avocado topped with balsamic vinegar 50g nuts (not peanuts) 1 Fat Bomb	6–8 glasses of water Tea and coffee (herbal or decaf if you prefer) In coffee and tea, try sticking with double cream or unsweetened almond or coconut milk

JOURNAL EXERCISE

You are now heading into Week Six of your Sugar Free journey and you're probably starting to think about your favourite meals and whether you will ever be able to eat them again. Remember that we are talking about a LCHF way of eating for life. With a few tweaks you should be able to keep many of your best-loved dishes in your meal plan – several of the recipes in this book have been adapted from some of my favourite meals.

Take a few minutes to write down a list of your favourite meals, meals that you could adapt for the LCHF way of eating. You may also want to spend some time searching on the internet to find similar recipes that fit in with the LCHF lifestyle. You could search for ketogenic dinners, paleo pizza, Banting ribs or LCHF bangers and mash. You could even do a search for low-carb sugar-free desserts (but avoid those recipes that have sugar substitutes).

Getting your family on the sugar-free, low-carb lifestyle

Here are some ideas of how to keep your children's food options both healthy and fun:

● Make your own food rules by giving your children last night's dinner leftovers for breakfast.
● Nuts and biltong are great for a snack on the go. They also make good lunchbox staples.
● Make cottage pie low carb by topping it with mashed sweet potato.

● Full-fat Greek yogurt can be sweetened with fruit.
● Blocks of cheese and apple make lovely skewers.
● Seed crackers (see recipe on page 215) can be topped with just about anything.
● Have cold meats available in the fridge.

Sugar Free does not have to be boring! Are you ready to invest in your children's health?

10   Love my body

Exercise is only one part of becoming body-healthy; we also need to love our bodies. As they are. It can be a difficult thing to do with the altered images presented to us in media and advertising. In Week Six we look at ways to help you get more in touch with your body and what it really needs.

Learning to love your body

What are we without our bodies? And yet how easy is it to take them for granted? The old adage 'your body is your temple' is very true. Our bodies are the vehicles through which we experience our external and internal worlds. However, many of us are consumed only by external appearances. We believe that fitting society's stereotypical image of beauty is the key to happiness and love.

We're bombarded daily with images and messages about what our physical appearance should be for us to be acceptable. We strive for the day we'll fit into a size 8, or when we finally have that thigh gap or whatever our ideal of physical perfection is. The truth is that striving for unattainable physical ideals leaves us feeling unwilling to accept our bodies as they are.

Comparing ourselves to others (or photoshopped media images) always results in one of two feelings: superiority or inferiority to the other person. Neither feeling is healthy, so our aim in recovery is to start learning to love and accept our bodies as they are.

Many of us also feel the need to 'pad' ourselves by using our bodies as shields from the outside world. Layers of fat are accumulated in the hope that we won't be hurt, shamed or embarrassed. Hiding behind our layers allows us to stay stuck in our addictive thought cycles of self-hate and fear, and to not have to take responsibility for ourselves. Our bodies bear the brunt of our binges, hateful thoughts and abusive behaviours. Would you treat someone else the way you've treated your body?

It's time for this abuse to stop, to start examining and mending this toxic relationship. But where do we start? I've found two of the greatest obstacles to loving and accepting our physical appearance are the scales and the mirror.

THE SCALES

To many of us the scales are an instrument of torture because they can severely limit our appreciation

   CHAPTER TEN

of our body – judging its amazing capabilities on a numerical value sounds ludicrous, yet it's what many of us do as soon as we wake up. That number on the scales will determine our mood: 80kg or more equals unhappiness, while 79kg or less equates to cheerfulness and excitement. Strange that one kilo can yield so much power.

THE MIRROR

Mirror, mirror on the wall, who's the prettiest of them all? This piece of glass can also become a form of punishment. Staring at your reflection, and searching for ways to beat yourself up, doesn't build self-esteem, self-love and self-acceptance.

Restore exercise

Depending on your relationship with these two inanimate yet powerful objects, I suggest you hide the scales and cover the mirror. Until you're able to start loving and appreciating yourself exactly as you are, I really do not want you to torture yourself.

It's time to redefine your own body concept by getting real. The chances are that if you are blessed with gorgeous childbearing hips and a curvaceous figure, you won't magically transform into the boyish shape popularised by catwalk models.

In order for us to start loving and accepting our bodies we need to start appreciating exactly what we have been blessed with. Stop wishing to be something you will never be and start loving your body as it is, knowing that 'upgrades' can be made with hard work, clean eating and exercise.

Now write a love letter to your body

The first step in re-establishing your relationship with your body is to bring awareness to it in a positive, gratitude-filled way. Instead of focusing on all the negative aspects of your body, start seeing it as a vehicle to your dreams. That's right, this body that's making you feel trapped holds the key to unlocking your true potential. As a first exercise, write a love letter to your body. It's been your constant companion since you were born, and will be with you until you die – isn't it time you showed a little love and appreciation?

Karen's Love Letter to her body

Dear Body

It seems we've been out of touch for a while. I'm sorry about the way I've been treating you. I've been filling you with junk and expecting you to be beautiful. Then when you don't live up to my ideals I punish you some more.

I'd like to make a promise to you that this will stop. I appreciate you and everything you do for me. Without you I wouldn't be able to live my life or have the experiences I've had. I wouldn't be able to hug my children or even sing a song. I wouldn't smell the wetness of the rain or feel sunlight on my skin.

My amazing body, I've taken you for granted. I'm now ready to create a long, happy and healthy relationship with you. It would be great if we could go for at least a 10-minute walk every day. I'd also like us to try different exercises such as running, yoga and horse riding.

When you're tired I'll make sure you get enough rest. When you're aching I will soak you in a hot bath. I'll rub lotion on you and start taking care of your external and internal needs. I commit to following my new lifestyle plan as I know it nourishes you on the inside and outside.

My dearest body, I see now that I've abused you badly and I'm truly sorry. I look forward to many more magical experiences with you. Thank you for not giving up on me.

With absolute love and gratitude

Karen

Journal exercise

Write your own love letter to your body. You may want to thank it for all its hard work over the years. Or perhaps apologise for how you've abused and misused it. Importantly, make a promise to your body that you'll start to look after it. Explain what you're going to do to restore your body and yourself to health.

CHAPTER TEN

First impressions

We create first impressions by how we dress, by the way we carry ourselves, and with the image we show the outside world. Does the image you project reflect the image you have of yourself as a dynamic/interesting/creative/funny/amazing person?

Ask yourself two other questions:

1 Do you dress in clothing that flatters your body shape and size or do you hide in baggy, shapeless clothing?
2 Do you feel confident and comfortable in how you present yourself to the outside world?

★

Tips for dealing with negative comments

Changing and experimenting with the way that you dress and present yourself to the outside world can be challenging and you won't always get it right. There's nothing more humiliating than trying a new 'look' and having somebody comment: 'You're not going out like that, are you?' Many of us will run straight to the kitchen cupboard in a desperate search for those long-lost Jelly Babies.

At times like these (and there will be), it's important to realise that what really matters is the way you feel about and see yourself. Remember Week Five's discussion about self-esteem and core beliefs? Don't allow other opinions of you to ruin your day.

When faced with a comment that shakes your self-esteem, take a few minutes to identify the feeling (shame, embarrassment or fear) and find a healthy outlet for it. Remind yourself of your positive core belief:

- I'm worthwhile
- I'm lovable
- I deserve to be treated with respect
- I accept myself as I am
- I have a right to express my feelings and emotions appropriately
- I am enough

Say it to yourself and believe it. If you do feel hurt by that person's words, think about telling them how it made you feel. People often say things without realising the impact their words can have. My husband always reminds me that what someone else thinks of me is none of my business.

Billy's story

I worked for a major restaurant chain for thirteen years after leaving school. During this phase of my life I ate a carb-rich diet and paid little regard to my increasing girth and failing health. I worked in London from 2001 until late 2005. It pushed my health and weight over the top. I was diagnosed as a type 2 diabetic but was in complete denial, so I carried on eating as before. I topped the scales at a massive 163kg and during a trip to Victoria Falls in July 2012 I received my wake-up call, chronically diabetic with extremely elevated blood pressure. I was at my wits' end and begged my GP for advice.

I discovered Professor Noakes on the internet and the lights went on. The simple fact was that carbs had taken me to this morbidly obese place and were keeping me there. All the previous diets I'd tried over the years had failed. Their common denominator? None of them cut out carbs completely.

Over the next twenty-eight weeks I lost over 80kg. During week sixteen, I lost 6.9kg in one week. The biggest cause of my dramatic weight loss was cutting my total carb intake to under 25g a day. Cravings? Oh yes! Initially I dreamt of bread. This lasted for about two weeks. Crutches? Oh yes! The gym became my crutch. The more weight I lost, the more I enjoyed going to the gym. During the first twenty-eight weeks, I rigidly followed an extremely low carb intake. I remember an early dream in which I ate bread. I awoke feeling mortified and guilty until I realised it was in my imagination. Initially it felt like my body was in detox, with headaches striking quite often. Nowadays, if I inadvertently eat any form of sugar, I immediately get a bad headache.

Most importantly, I've been off all diabetes medication at the advice of my GP since the beginning of 2013. My lifestyle change is part of who I am now. It defines my choices when eating out, when I shop and during socialising.

Low carb is part of my life. I don't find it difficult to follow. It gave me back my life and I will be eternally grateful to Professor Tim Noakes and all the other brave pioneers out there, who persevere in exploding the food pyramid myth in the face of harsh and undue criticism. Their work saves lives.

WEEKLY JOURNAL EXERCISE

Take a few minutes to reflect on your week and this stage of your journey:

1. What were your greatest successes this week?
2. How will you build on your successes?
3. Did you stick to your meal plan?
4. Did you maintain abstinence from sugar and carbs?
5. If not, what triggered you to relapse or slip? What have you learnt from this experience?
6. What exercise did you do this week?
7. Are you unhappy about anything that happened this week?
8. Have you been affirming yourself?
9. What will you do differently next week to support your journey in recovery positively?
10. Make a list of ten things you are grateful for.

Affirmation
I am so grateful for the body I have. I choose to treat it with love and respect.

USEFUL RESOURCES

Women, Food and God: An Unexpected Path to Almost Everything by Geneen Roth (Simon & Schuster Ltd, 2011). What you eat is inseparable from your core beliefs about being alive. This is an intimate portrayal of our need for thinness and the supposed happiness and acceptance that comes with it. Geneen Roth identifies what weight loss and dieting really mean in a journey towards healing.

Mindful Eating: A Guide to Rediscovering a Healthy and Joyful Relationship with Food by Jan Chozen Bays (Shambala Publications, 2009). The art of mindfulness can transform our struggle with food – and renew our sense of pleasure, appreciation and satisfaction with eating.

DAY 36

Breakfast	Lunch	Dinner	Snacks	Drinks
Green Smoothie (see recipe)	3 Scrambled eggs with 3 slices (60g) pre-cooked ham, ¼ of a courgette and 6 cherry tomatoes	Chicken Aubergine 'Lasagne' (see recipe; keep some for tomorrow) served with a green salad dressed with olive oil	**Consume up to 2 snacks per day and only when hungry** 10 olives Up to 30g hard cheese 10 Parmesan Crisps with 1 tbsp homemade Guacamole or homemade salsa ½ an avocado topped with balsamic vinegar 50g nuts (not peanuts) 1 Fat Bomb	6–8 glasses of water Tea and coffee (herbal or decaf if you prefer) In coffee and tea, try sticking with double cream or unsweetened almond or coconut milk

DAY 37

Breakfast	Lunch	Dinner	Snacks	Drinks
Greek-style omelette made with 3 eggs, 40g feta cheese, 1tsp dried basil and ½ tsp dried oregano 10 olives and 6 cherry tomatoes topped with fresh coriander	Creamy Avocado Soup (see recipe) with 1 or 2 seed crackers	Chicken Aubergine 'Lasagne' (left over from last night's dinner) served with a green salad dressed with olive oil	**Consume up to 2 snacks per day and only when hungry** 10 olives Up to 30g hard cheese 10 Parmesan Crisps with 1 tbsp homemade Guacamole or homemade salsa ½ an avocado topped with balsamic vinegar 50g nuts (not peanuts) 1 Fat Bomb	6–8 glasses of water Tea and coffee (herbal or decaf if you prefer) In coffee and tea, try sticking with double cream or unsweetened almond or coconut milk

DAY 38

Breakfast	Lunch	Dinner	Snacks	Drinks
3 tbsp natural whole-milk (or Greek) yogurt mixed with 1 tbsp double cream (optional), 1 tbsp coconut flakes, 30g mixed nuts and 50g berries	Spiced omelette: 3 large eggs whisked with 4 tsp milk or double cream, finely chopped onion and red pepper, coriander, cumin and ½–1 tsp chilli powder. Serve with fresh salad or guacamole	Chilli con Carne (see recipe; keep some for tomorrow) with Cauliflower Rice (see recipe)	**Consume up to 2 snacks per day and only when hungry** 10 olives Up to 30g hard cheese 10 Parmesan Crisps with 1 tbsp homemade Guacamole or homemade salsa ½ an avocado topped with balsamic vinegar 50g nuts (not peanuts) 1 Fat Bomb	6–8 glasses of water Tea and coffee (herbal or decaf if you prefer) In coffee and tea, try sticking with double cream or unsweetened almond or coconut milk

Breakfast	Lunch	Dinner	Snacks	Drinks
3 rashers of bacon with 50g cream cheese and 50g berries	Caprese Salad (see recipe)	Chilli con Carne (left over from last night's dinner) with Cauliflower Rice (see recipe)	**Consume up to 2 snacks per day and only when hungry** 10 olives Up to 30g hard cheese 10 Parmesan Crisps with 1 tbsp homemade Guacamole or homemade salsa ½ an avocado topped with balsamic vinegar 50g nuts (not peanuts) 1 Fat Bomb	6–8 glasses of water Tea and coffee (herbal or decaf if you prefer) In coffee and tea, try sticking with double cream or unsweetened almond or coconut milk

Breakfast	Lunch	Dinner	Snacks	Drinks
3tbsp natural whole-milk (or Greek) yogurt mixed with (50g) sugar-free Nut Granola (see recipe) and 50g berries	Chicken and bacon salad: up to 100g chicken and 50g bacon with 3 handfuls of salad leaves, 50g cucumber and 8 cherry tomatoes, with olive oil and cider vinegar dressing	Salmon fillet (grilled, baked or fried) topped with 1tbsp homemade green pesto, served with 3 grilled vine tomatoes and 8 spears of asparagus (served with butter)	**Consume up to 2 snacks per day and only when hungry** 10 olives Up to 30g hard cheese 10 Parmesan Crisps with 1 tbsp homemade Guacamole or homemade salsa ½ an avocado topped with balsamic vinegar 50g nuts (not peanuts) 1 Fat Bomb	6–8 glasses of water Tea and coffee (herbal or decaf if you prefer) In coffee and tea, try sticking with double cream or unsweetened almond or coconut milk

Breakfast	Lunch	Dinner	Snacks	Drinks
2 eggs (cooked any way you like), 3 rashers of bacon, 1 good-quality sausage (at least 80% meat), 1 flat mushroom	Thai Green Curry	2 grilled lamb chops served with 2 portions of vegetables	**Consume up to 2 snacks per day and only when hungry** 10 olives Up to 30g hard cheese 10 Parmesan Crisps with 1 tbsp homemade Guacamole or homemade salsa ½ an avocado topped with balsamic vinegar 50g nuts (not peanuts) 1 Fat Bomb	6–8 glasses of water Tea and coffee (herbal or decaf if you prefer) In coffee and tea, try sticking with double cream or unsweetened almond or coconut milk

Breakfast	Lunch	Dinner	Snacks	Drinks
2 Egg and Parma Ham Cups (see recipe) served with 1 tbsp sour cream	Super Green Soup (see recipe) served with 1 slice Nut and Seed Loaf (see recipe)	1 medium-steak (about 150g) with garlic butter and roasted celeriac (50g uncooked weight) and sweet potato chips (50g uncooked weight)	**Consume up to 2 snacks per day and only when hungry** 10 olives Up to 30g hard cheese 10 Parmesan Crisps with 1 tbsp homemade Guacamole or homemade salsa ½ an avocado topped with balsamic vinegar 50g nuts (not peanuts) 1 Fat Bomb	6–8 glasses of water Tea and coffee (herbal or decaf if you prefer) In coffee and tea, try sticking with double cream or unsweetened almond or coconut milk

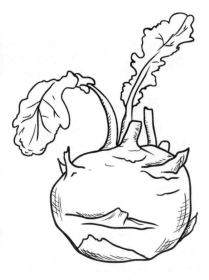

　　CHAPTER TEN

Breakfast	Lunch	Dinner	Snacks	Drinks
3 tbsp natural whole-milk (or Greek) yogurt mixed with 50g sugar free granola	Warm goat's cheese and walnut salad: 50g goat's cheese (heated under the grill for 5 minutes), 30g walnuts, 2 large handfuls of young spinach leaves, 1 handful of rocket, ½ a green pepper, 50g cucumber, with olive oil and cider vinegar dressing (3 parts oil to 1 vinegar)	2 slices of low-carb pizza, served with Celeriac Chips (see recipe)	**Consume up to 2 snacks per day and only when hungry** 10 olives Up to 30g hard cheese ½ an avocado topped with balsamic vinegar 50g nuts (not peanuts) 1 Fat Bomb	6–8 glasses of water Tea and coffee (herbal or decaf if you prefer) In coffee and tea, try sticking with double cream or unsweetened almond or coconut milk

Breakfast	Lunch	Dinner	Snacks	Drinks
Egg 'muffins': whisk together 4 eggs, chopped tomato, green pepper and onion. Pour into buttered muffin tins and fill halfway. Bake in the oven at 160°C for 15 minutes or until cooked	Grilled halloumi salad: 60g halloumi, 2 large handfuls of young spinach leaves, 1 handful of rocket, ½ a green pepper, 50g cucumber, with olive oil and cider vinegar dressing (3 parts oil to 1 vinegar)	Aubergine 'pizzas': cut aubergine into 1cm discs (up to 8 slices), spread with sun-dried tomato paste, top with a slice of mozzarella and a slice of Cheddar cheese and sprinkle with basil. Grill for 5–10 minutes. Serve with sautéed spinach	**Consume up to 2 snacks per day and only when hungry** 10 olives Up to 30g hard cheese ½ an avocado topped with balsamic vinegar 50g nuts (not peanuts) 1 Fat Bomb	6–8 glasses of water Tea and coffee (herbal or decaf if you prefer) In coffee and tea, try sticking with double cream or unsweetened almond or coconut milk

Breakfast	Lunch	Dinner	Snacks	Drinks
Warm Chia Seed Breakfast Mug (see recipe)	Beetroot and goat's cheese salad: 50g goat's cheese, 50g diced fresh beetroot, 30g walnuts, 2 large handfuls of young spinach leaves, 1 handful of rocket, ½ a green pepper, 50g cucumber, with olive oil and cider vinegar dressing (3 parts oil to 1 vinegar)	Mushroom Stroganoff (see recipe; keep some for tomorrow) with Cauliflower Rice (see recipe)	**Consume up to 2 snacks per day and only when hungry** 10 olives Up to 30g hard cheese ½ an avocado topped with balsamic vinegar 50g nuts (not peanuts) 1 Fat Bomb	6–8 glasses of water Tea and coffee (herbal or decaf if you prefer) In coffee and tea, try sticking with double cream or unsweetened almond or coconut milk

Breakfast	Lunch	Dinner	Snacks	Drinks
Egg and avocado platter: 3 eggs (cooked any way you like) ½ an avocado and 6 cherry tomatoes	2 slices of of Cauliflower Pizza with a large salad	Mushroom Stroganoff (see recipe; left over from last night's dinner) with Cauliflower Rice	**Consume up to 2 snacks per day and only when hungry** 10 olives Up to 30g hard cheese ½ an avocado topped with balsamic vinegar 50g nuts (not peanuts) 1 Fat Bomb	6–8 glasses of water Tea and coffee (herbal or decaf if you prefer) In coffee and tea, try sticking with double cream or unsweetened almond or coconut milk

Breakfast	Lunch	Dinner	Snacks	Drinks
3 tbsp natural whole-milk (or Greek) yogurt with 50g of sugar-free Nut Granola (see recipe)	Grilled halloumi salad: up to 60g halloumi, 2 large handfuls of young spinach leaves, 1 handful of rocket, ½ a green pepper, 50g cucumber, with olive oil and cider vinegar dressing (3 parts oil to 1 vinegar)	Spinach and Courgette Burgers (see recipe) topped with Cheddar cheese and served with a large salad drizzled with olive oil	**Consume up to 2 snacks per day and only when hungry** 10 olives Up to 30g hard cheese ½ an avocado topped with balsamic vinegar 50g nuts (not peanuts) 1 Fat Bomb	6–8 glasses of water Tea and coffee (herbal or decaf if you prefer) In coffee and tea, try sticking with double cream or unsweetened almond or coconut milk

Breakfast	Lunch	Dinner	Snacks	Drinks
Egg and avocado platter: 3 eggs (cooked any way you like) and ½ an avocado (those not as sensitive to sugar can add 6 cherry tomatoes)	Green Soup (see recipe)	Cauliflower Mac 'n' Cheese Bake (see recipe) served with a large salad dressed with olive oil	**Consume up to 2 snacks per day and only when hungry** 10 olives Up to 30g hard cheese ½ an avocado topped with balsamic vinegar 50g nuts (not peanuts) 1 Fat Bomb	6–8 glasses of water Tea and coffee (herbal or decaf if you prefer) In coffee and tea, try sticking with double cream or unsweetened almond or coconut milk

Breakfast	Lunch	Dinner	Snacks	Drinks
3 tbsp natural whole-milk (or Greek) yogurt mixed with 1 tbsp double cream (optional), 1 tbsp coconut flakes, 30g mixed nuts and 50g berries	1 Mocha Protein Smoothie (see recipe)	Stuffed aubergine (see recipe)	**Consume up to 2 snacks per day and only when hungry** 10 olives Up to 30g hard cheese ½ an avocado topped with balsamic vinegar 50g nuts (not peanuts) 1 Fat Bomb	6–8 glasses of water Tea and coffee (herbal or decaf if you prefer) In coffee and tea, try sticking with double cream or unsweetened almond or coconut milk

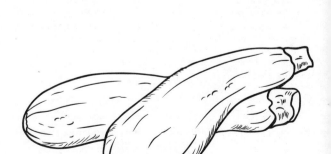

11   Cultivating mindfulness

The eight-
week plan
Week 7

Adult human beings have astounding brains – we have an average of 100 billion neurons that create nearly 10,000 synaptic connections to other neurons. That's over three million kilometres of neural highway – in our brains. You can get dizzy just thinking about it.

Our brains are wired in this way to process incalculable amounts of information every millisecond – your brain is processing what you're seeing, hearing, smelling, tasting, touching and sensing, and it can do this all at the same time. It's not surprising, therefore, that sometimes it's difficult to turn our brains off or focus our attention on only one thing.

Who hasn't has been in a situation where your mind races ahead so much that you aren't paying attention to what's being said and miss the punchline of the joke – and then wonder why everyone else is laughing. Or you've driven home on automatic pilot and can't remember whether the traffic lights were red or green?

Wouldn't it be wonderful if there were a way to tap into the spectacular nature of the world, moment by moment? A way to remind ourselves of its beauty? A way to slow down to appreciate important things happening around us: a blackbird singing on a summer evening; the first steps of a child; the warmth of the sun; connecting to other people in a real and meaningful way.

Practising mindfulness is a way to do this. Mindfulness is simply paying attention to the present moment in a conscious way. When being mindful you're also non-judgemental towards yourself and other people.

Why mindfulness is so important in the process of recovery
As addicts we may have lost contact with our bodies and ourselves – we don't face ourselves in the mirror, and we ignore the loving, kind thoughts we should have about ourselves. When in full addict behaviour we're not paying attention to ourselves or the people and world around us. Our mind races in a hundred different directions – we find it hard to keep focused on our recovery. We tend to ruminate on a negative thought until it's blown out of proportion. We end up 'living in our heads'.

Mindfulness helps you get to know your mind and bring it under control. When being mindful you're not trying to change anything –

you're simply paying attention to your mind, and when you do that it starts to calm down. Think about children when they're fractious and noisy – when you really pay attention to them and listen they'll often calm down. When last did you take time out and really pay attention to yourself?

Restore exercise

Take a few minutes to practise mindfulness right now:

● Sit on the edge of your chair so that your spine is upright and both feet are on the floor.
Just focus on your breathing – in and out, in and out.
● Bring your attention to your belly – you may want to put your hand there.
● Now imagine there is a light or candle in your belly.
● Put your mind into that light or candle.
● Just breathe in and out, in and out. When your mind wanders, say something loving and kind to yourself: 'Ah, there goes my mind again?' or 'Now there's a thought'.

Mindfulness and your critical voice

As addicts we often have a critical voice in our heads telling us we're ugly or fat or not good enough, or that no one loves us. It's easy to get caught up in what that voice is telling us, and to stop paying attention to the world around us. We begin ruminating on negative thoughts.

By practising mindfulness in that moment, we can shift our way of thinking. It's not about banishing the voice or being critical towards it – it's simply about placing your attention somewhere else (usually on your breath) and acknowledging that voice with words of love and kindness.

You're not trying to change anything by being mindful. You're simply paying attention to what's happening in that moment. Mindfulness is something that requires effort and focus. Our minds are so used to non-mindful practice that they resist change. That's why we encourage you to be gentle and kind with yourself. Find a mindfulness practice that works for you and do it consistently.

Here are some suggestions:
● Take a mindful walk by yourself once a week. When you're walking, use all your senses to tune in to the world around you.
● Identify a daily habit that you can change into a mindful practice – washing the dishes or brushing your teeth. Pay attention to what you're doing. If you feel your mind is wandering then gently bring it back to your activity.
● Spend five minutes every day focusing on your breathing.

Once you're comfortable with a simple mindfulness practice you may want to consider learning to meditate. Have a look at the resources on p141, or download my guided meditations from thesugarfreerevolution.com.

Journal exercise

How easy or difficult did you find the Restore exercise? Did you find your mind racing to other thoughts? How did you bring back your attention to your breathing? Were you non-judgemental? Did you say something loving and kind to yourself when your mind wandered?

Karen

During my recovery I developed a habit of checking my email and social media last thing before I fell asleep and as soon as I woke up. I became preoccupied with what was happening outside myself. I'd slipped into a very bad habit that was addictive in nature.

My days became rushed because immediately after reading my email my mind started racing about everything that needed to be done. I started worrying and living in the future, with unfounded fears and worries. My monkey mind was out of control – I woke up in the middle of the night realising I was moving further and further from my recovery and myself. It scared me. So I made a conscious decision to always start and end my day in exactly the same way. No matter where I am, this routine keeps me grounded.

Now I wake up at least 30 minutes before I need to get my kids up for school. I sit in a quiet, peaceful place and breathe. I dedicate this quiet time to myself. I use the time to set my intentions for the day. Once I feel peaceful and calm, I make myself coffee, get breakfast ready and wake up the kids. My morning ritual allows me to lay a foundation that carries me through the busyness of my day.

My ritual at night had me going back to basics. Every night I write ten things that I'm grateful for and I write my affirmation ten times. I also say a prayer of gratitude and acknowledgement to my higher power. I then listen to a guided meditation (my current favourite is Deepak Chopra: chopra.com/ccl/guided-meditations). Regardless of what happens I try to start and finish my day by being mindful.

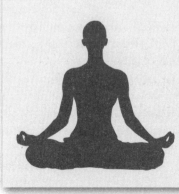

★

Tips for managing buffets

At some point you'll be confronted with a situation where food is freely available – this could be a buffet at a wedding or a snack table at an event. When confronted with a large amount of food, your urge to overeat and also to eat sugar and carbs could become overwhelming. The important thing is to eat slowly and mindfully. Be conscious about your food choices and what you are putting into your mouth.

These techniques will help you:

● Use a small plate.

● Only cover 80 per cent of your plate's surface with food. Don't pile foods on top of each other. Stick to healthy food choices.

● Take one bite and really taste the food.

● Chew slowly. Savour the taste and texture of what you're eating.

● If you're eating with a knife and fork, put down your cutlery while chewing your food.

● If you're standing and eating, put the finger food back on your plate while you're chewing.

● Only once you've chewed at least twenty times, take the next bite of food.

● When you've finished your plate, don't immediately rush to fill it.

● Take time to enjoy the conversation around you. If after 20 minutes you still feel hungry, then return to the buffet.

● Only fill 20 per cent of your plate's surface this time. Stick to healthy food choices.

● When you eat, savour each mouthful. Put down your cutlery or piece of food in between bites.

The important thing is to eat slowly and mindfully. Be conscious about your food choices and what you are putting into your mouth.

Kobus's story

I've always been able to maintain my weight within reasonable limits. But once I hit my early fifties I experienced a gradual increase in my weight, to such an extent that my clothes became undersized and I could feel I was fatter. I increased my exercise rate, but it had hardly any significant influence on weight loss.

Towards the latter half of 2012 I became aware of a number of discussions around the merits of increasing fat and decreasing carbohydrates in your diet. It's a debate that intrigued me. I decided to give it a try.

All the advice and information proposed in the LCHF plan went directly against the thinking that had been 'drilled' into us over decades. Presentations by Professor Tim Noakes and Swedish medical doctor Andreas Eenfeldt, and learning from the success stories I observed at the HELP Program, persuaded me sufficiently to attempt this 'radical' eating plan. I was hesitant, especially with the outcry from certain corners in the medical profession. But I admire Prof. Noakes for not being bullied by a strong lobbying fraternity in that profession.

I've followed my own broad plan in sugar and carbohydrate reduction. At the end of 2013 I stopped eating bread, pasta and pizza, potato and rice products, and chocolates. At the same time I started enjoying the crispy fat on lamb chops, having more eggs and bacon, switching from low-fat to full-cream milk, and indulging in cheese and lots of green vegetables.

My weight went from 100kg to 95kg. I didn't feel as hungry as I used to; my usual craving for something sweet was greatly reduced, almost nullified. As time went on, I lost more weight and now weigh 88kg. I exercise moderately for cardiovascular purposes and not to lose weight. I've maintained my weight between 88kg and 90kg for over a year. I feel good within myself and my 'grazing' has stopped.

LCHF produces results with relatively little physical effort. Apart from being in better physical shape, I have an improved state of mind; weight loss affects a person's demeanour. In addition, I'd been on statins for twenty years and I've now stopped using them altogether.

WEEKLY JOURNAL EXERCISE

Take a few minutes to reflect on your week and this stage of your journey:

1. What were your greatest successes this week?
2. How will you build on your successes?
3. Did you stick to your meal plan?
4. Did you maintain abstinence from sugar and carbs?
5. If not, what triggered you to relapse or slip? What have you learnt from this experience?
6. What exercise did you do this week?
7. Are you unhappy about anything that happened this week?
8. Have you been affirming yourself?
9. What will you do differently next week to support your journey in recovery positively?
10. Make a list of ten things you are grateful for.

♥

Affirmation
I am content
right here
and now.

USEFUL RESOURCES

Sane New World: Taming the Mind by Ruby Wax (Hodder & Stoughton, 2013). Comedian and mental health campaigner Ruby Wax has a funny take on mental illness. Her book provides information about how the brain malfunctions in mental illness, tells her own story, and offers many tips and exercises for practising mindfulness.

Turning the Mind into an Ally by Sakyong Mipham (Riverhead Books, 2003). One of the best books on meditation and on the nature of the mind, written by a leading Tibetan Buddhist teacher. Having grown up in America, Sakyong Mipham relates to and tells stories from a western cultural perspective.

DAY 43

Breakfast	Lunch	Dinner	Snacks	Drinks
3 tbsp natural whole-milk yogurt with 50g of sugar-free Nut Granola (see recipe)	Salmon (100–120g uncooked) fillet, baked or grilled, with 1tbsp homemade pesto, served with 2 portions of vegetables	Philly Steak Stuffed Mushrooms (see recipe) with a large side salad	**Consume up to 2 snacks per day and only when hungry** 10 olives Up to 30g hard cheese 10 Parmesan Crisps with 1 tbsp homemade Guacamole or homemade salsa ½ an avocado topped with balsamic vinegar 50g nuts (not peanuts) 1 Fat Bomb	6–8 glasses of water Tea and coffee (herbal or decaf if you prefer) In coffee and tea, try sticking with double cream or unsweetened almond or coconut milk

DAY 44

Breakfast	Lunch	Dinner	Snacks	Drinks
2 eggs (scrambled, fried, boiled) with 2–3 rashers of bacon and ½ an avocado	Mini Salami Pizzas (see recipe) with a large side salad dressed with olive oil and cider vinegar	Pork Stroganoff (see recipe; keep some for tomorrow) with Cauliflower Rice.	**Consume up to 2 snacks per day and only when hungry** 10 olives Up to 30g hard cheese 10 Parmesan Crisps with 1 tbsp homemade Guacamole or homemade salsa ½ an avocado topped with balsamic vinegar 50g nuts (not peanuts) 1 Fat Bomb	6–8 glasses of water Tea and coffee (herbal or decaf if you prefer) In coffee and tea, try sticking with double cream or unsweetened almond or coconut milk

DAY 45

Breakfast	Lunch	Dinner	Snacks	Drinks
2–3 eggs scrambled with 2tbsp double cream, 1 handful of chives and spinach served with 50g of salmon – optional	Salad (salad leaves, cucumber, peppers, tomatoes, celery) with any protein option (around 100 –150g) with lemon and olive oil dressing – can also sprinkle some seeds on top	Pork Stroganoff (left over from last night's dinner) with Cauliflower Rice (see recipe)	**Consume up to 2 snacks per day and only when hungry** 10 olives Up to 30g hard cheese 10 Parmesan Crisps with 1 tbsp homemade Guacamole or homemade salsa ½ an avocado topped with balsamic vinegar 50g nuts (not peanuts) 1 Fat Bomb	6–8 glasses of water Tea and coffee (herbal or decaf if you prefer) In coffee and tea, try sticking with double cream or unsweetened almond or coconut milk

Breakfast	Lunch	Dinner	Snacks	Drinks
Warm Chia Seed Breakfast Mug (see recipe)	Chorizo (up to 50g), red pepper and goats' cheese (30g) 2–3 egg omelette	Creamy Mushroom and Ham 'Pasta' (see recipe)	**Consume up to 2 snacks per day and only when hungry** 10 olives Up to 30g hard cheese 10 Parmesan Crisps with 1 tbsp homemade Guacamole or homemade salsa ½ an avocado topped with balsamic vinegar 50g nuts (not peanuts) 1 Fat Bomb	6–8 glasses of water Tea and coffee (herbal or decaf if you prefer) In coffee and tea, try sticking with double cream or unsweetened almond or coconut milk

Breakfast	Lunch	Dinner	Snacks	Drinks
Egg, salmon and avocado platter: 3 eggs (cooked any way you like), 50g salmon (any kind) ½ an avocado and 6 cherry tomatoes	Steak (100g uncooked weight) and blue cheese salad: (up to 30g cheese), 1 handful of young spinach leaves, 1 handful of rocket, ½ green pepper, 50g cucumber, 3 celery stalks	2 large flat mushrooms stuffed with mozzarella, topped with herbs of your choice and grilled, served with 2 portions of vegetables	**Consume up to 2 snacks per day and only when hungry** 10 olives Up to 30g hard cheese 10 Parmesan Crisps with 1 tbsp homemade Guacamole or homemade salsa ½ an avocado topped with balsamic vinegar 50g nuts (not peanuts) 1 Fat Bomb	6–8 glasses of water Tea and coffee (herbal or decaf if you prefer) In coffee and tea, try sticking with double cream or unsweetened almond or coconut milk

Breakfast	Lunch	Dinner	Snacks	Drinks
3 tbsp natural whole-milk yogurt with 50g sugar free Nut Granola (see recipe)	Salad (salad leaves, cucumber, peppers, tomatoes, celery) with any protein option (around 100–150g) with lemon and olive oil dressing – can also sprinkle some seeds on top	Lamb Koftas (see recipe) served with a small Greek salad and 1tbsp of crème fraîche	**Consume up to 2 snacks per day and only when hungry** 10 olives Up to 30g hard cheese 10 Parmesan Crisps with 1 tbsp homemade Guacamole or homemade salsa ½ an avocado topped with balsamic vinegar 50g nuts (not peanuts) 1 Fat Bomb	6–8 glasses of water Tea and coffee (herbal or decaf if you prefer) In coffee and tea, try sticking with double cream or unsweetened almond or coconut milk

Breakfast	Lunch	Dinner	Snacks	Drinks
Berry Smoothie (see recipe)	3 eggs scrambled with 2 handfuls of shredded spinach, 1 handful of chopped spring onions and 1 tbsp grated Parmesan, served with homemade salsa and a large salad	Chicken parmesan then roasted for 20 mins at 180°C, served with 100g green beans and 100g mushrooms cooked in butter	**Consume up to 2 snacks per day and only when hungry** 10 olives Up to 30g hard cheese 10 Parmesan Crisps with 1 tbsp homemade Guacamole or homemade salsa ½ an avocado topped with balsamic vinegar 50g nuts (not peanuts) 1 Fat Bomb	6–8 glasses of water Tea and coffee (herbal or decaf if you prefer) In coffee and tea, try sticking with double cream or unsweetened almond or coconut milk

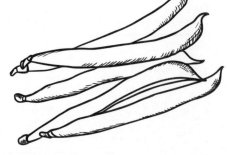

Breakfast	Lunch	Dinner	Snacks	Drinks
3 tbsp natural whole-milk (or Greek) yogurt mixed with 1 tbsp double cream (optional), 1 tbsp coconut flakes, 30g mixed nuts and 50g berries	Salad of rocket, spinach, black and green olives and up to 50g feta cheese with olive oil and vinegar dressing	Cheesy Courgette 'Pasta' (see recipe)	**Consume up to 2 snacks per day and only when hungry** 10 olives Up to 30g hard cheese ½ an avocado topped with balsamic vinegar 50g nuts (not peanuts) 1 Fat Bomb	6–8 glasses of water Tea and coffee (herbal or decaf if you prefer) In coffee and tea, try sticking with double cream or unsweetened almond or coconut milk

Breakfast	Lunch	Dinner	Snacks	Drinks
Warm Chia Seed Breakfast Mug (see recipe)	Green Smoothie (see recipe) with 3 celery stalks and almond butter	Coconut Camembert with Berry Salad (see recipe)	**Consume up to 2 snacks per day and only when hungry** 10 olives Up to 30g hard cheese ½ an avocado topped with balsamic vinegar 50g nuts (not peanuts) 1 Fat Bomb	6–8 glasses of water Tea and coffee (herbal or decaf if you prefer) In coffee and tea, try sticking with double cream or unsweetened almond or coconut milk

Breakfast	Lunch	Dinner	Snacks	Drinks
3 eggs scrambled with 3 chopped spring onions, 1 large handful of shredded spinach and some snipped chives	Beetroot and goat's cheese salad: 50g goat's cheese, 50g diced fresh beetroot, 30g walnuts, 2 large handfuls of young spinach leaves, 1 handful of rocket, ½ a green pepper, 50g cucumber, with olive oil and cider vinegar dressing (3 parts oil to 1 vinegar)	2 large mushrooms stuffed with mozzarella and ricotta cheese, and herbs of your choice, and grilled served with a large salad	**Consume up to 2 snacks per day and only when hungry** 10 olives Up to 30g hard cheese ½ an avocado topped with balsamic vinegar 50g nuts (not peanuts) 1 Fat Bomb	6–8 glasses of water Tea and coffee (herbal or decaf if you prefer) In coffee and tea, try sticking with double cream or unsweetened almond or coconut milk

Breakfast	Lunch	Dinner	Snacks	Drinks
3 tbsp natural whole-milk yogurt mixed with 1 tbsp almond butter, 1 tbsp coconut flakes, 30g mixed nuts and seeds and 50g berries	Green Smoothie (see recipe) with 3 celery stalks and almond butter	Baked Eggs with Asparagus and Mozzarella (see recipe)	**Consume up to 2 snacks per day and only when hungry** 10 olives Up to 30g hard cheese ½ an avocado topped with balsamic vinegar 50g nuts (not peanuts) 1 Fat Bomb	6–8 glasses of water Tea and coffee (herbal or decaf if you prefer) In coffee and tea, try sticking with double cream or unsweetened almond or coconut milk

Breakfast	Lunch	Dinner	Snacks	Drinks
Spiced omelette: 3 large eggs whisked with 4 tsp milk or double cream, finely chopped onion and red pepper, coriander, cumin and ½–1 tsp chilli powder. Serve with fresh salad or guacamole	Grilled halloumi salad: up to 60g halloumi with 2 large handfuls of young spinach leaves, 1 handful of rocket, ½ a green pepper, 50g cucumber, with olive oil and cider vinegar dressing (3 parts oil to 1 vinegar)	Aubergine 'pizzas': cut aubergine into 1cm discs (up to 8 slices), spread with sun-dried tomato paste, top with a slice of mozzarella and a slice of Cheddar cheese and sprinkle basil on top. Grill for 5–10 minutes. Serve with sautéed spinach	**Consume up to 2 snacks per day and only when hungry** 10 olives Up to 30g hard cheese ½ an avocado topped with balsamic vinegar 50g nuts (not peanuts) 1 Fat Bomb	6–8 glasses of water Tea and coffee (herbal or decaf if you prefer) In coffee and tea, try sticking with double cream or unsweetened almond or coconut milk

Breakfast	Lunch	Dinner	Snacks	Drinks
3 tbsp natural whole-milk (or Greek) yogurt mixed with 1 tbsp double cream (optional), 1 tbsp coconut flakes, 30g mixed nuts and 50g berries	Super Green Soup (see recipe)	Cauliflower Mushroom Risotto (see recipe) Parmesan cheese	**Consume up to 2 snacks per day and only when hungry** 10 olives Up to 30g hard cheese ½ an avocado topped with balsamic vinegar 50g nuts (not peanuts) 1 Fat Bomb	6–8 glasses of water Tea and coffee (herbal or decaf if you prefer) In coffee and tea, try sticking with double cream or unsweetened almond or coconut milk

CHAPTER ELEVEN

Breakfast	Lunch	Dinner	Snacks	Drinks
Berry Smoothie (see recipe)	Egg 'muffins': whisk together 4 eggs, chopped tomato, green pepper and onion. Pour into buttered muffin tins and fill halfway. Bake in the oven at 160°C for 15 minutes or until cooked	One red pepper stuffed with mushrooms and spinach creamed together with 50mls of double cream and 1tsp of butter, baked with 50g of mozzarella and 50g feta cheese for 10 minutes at 180°C	**Consume up to 2 snacks per day and only when hungry** 10 olives Up to 30g hard cheese ½ an avocado topped with balsamic vinegar 50g nuts (not peanuts) 1 Fat Bomb	6–8 glasses of water Tea and coffee (herbal or decaf if you prefer) In coffee and tea, try sticking with double cream or unsweetened almond or coconut milk

12 Relapse

The eight-
week plan
....
Week 8
....

Nobody is perfect. Sometimes we relapse. This doesn't mean you're stupid, have no willpower or will never stay 'clean'. It just means you had a relapse. During Week Eight we're exploring ways to recover from a relapse, no matter how big.

There will be times when even the most vigilant people can't resist the temptation of sugar and carbs. Often during intense emotional turmoil our resolve to stay clean is overridden by a deep desire to self-soothe with our external 'fix'. Addiction is a disease of relapse. The truth is that relapses happen. That isn't to say you should use a relapse as an excuse to binge or eat sugar or carbs. What we're saying is that should it happen it's what you do to get back on track that's important.

When you have a relapse the key thing to remember is: don't

Karen

One day a while back I went through a really tough time emotionally. I had immense feelings of anger and resentment towards my husband. My feelings overwhelmed and devastated me. I felt out of control emotionally and the only 'fix' I craved was to drown my sorrows with a bowl of pasta, followed by a cola, half a packet of biscuits and a bag of sweets, then wash it down with a sweetened cappuccino.

I entered a dream-like state of inebriation. I just wanted to sleep. I woke up in the middle of the night with a pounding headache and in desperate need of water. I overslept the next morning and woke up with what I can only describe as a hangover. Once this heroin-like dream state had passed, I realised I'd taken out on myself all the anger and resentment I'd felt towards my husband.

It took three days for my body to recover, and intense journaling to sort out my anger and resentment. If I'd thought those foods would fix my emotional state I was sadly mistaken.

beat yourself up. Try to find the lesson in your experience, and move on from there. A relapse isn't only caused by negative feelings. Often, celebrations such as birthday parties, promotions and house-warmings can prove to be our greatest challenges. Times of celebration have become synonymous with cakes, sweets and treats, often being forced upon us by well-meaning hosts. You'll often be confronted by suggestions such as 'You have to try this cake; I baked it myself', or 'Just have one biscuit; I could never deprive myself like that' when you refuse sugar and carbs at a celebration. Remember Week One when you were identifying ways to say no to sugar? No is a complete sentence.

Sometimes saying no when everyone else is saying yes – and seems to be having such a lovely time – can lead to feelings of deprivation. In times like these it's very important to remember that you've made a conscious choice not to eat sugar or carbs. You've done it because it benefits your health and wellbeing not only physically, but emotionally, mentally and spiritually too.

When you're struggling with these feelings of deprivation, take a minute to remind yourself why you're choosing not to fill your body with sugar and carbs. And if you can't do that exercise mentally, then rather excuse yourself, get some fresh air and a clearer perspective.

Relapses can be unconscious. Take Nadia:

Nadia's story

I was attending a catered event, and having a good time chatting and talking to people at my table. By the time dessert arrived I wasn't thinking about food. I was only thinking about what a good time I was having. I ate the dessert – a delicious lemon meringue pie – without thinking. I saw my neighbour had left half her pie and I asked her if she was going to finish it. She wasn't, so I ate that as well. Only when I put that last forkful into my mouth did I realise what I'd done.

Whenever you have a relapse, whether it's unconscious or conscious, it's important to keep the bigger picture in mind. That's even more crucial when you're feeling vulnerable, deprived and isolated. Saying 'What the hell, I've blown it so I may as well continue' will be tempting. Instead we suggest playing through your own addiction movie.

Play your own addiction movie
Sit back and lose the popcorn – this is an amazing opportunity to see your own addiction movie. You don't have to relapse to do this simple visualisation exercise; you can do it at any time.

A few simple questions to get you started:

- What are you favourite binge or cheat foods?
- Where do you like to eat them?

Now imagine you're in a supermarket shopping for food. Perhaps you've just had a fight with your boss/husband/girlfriend/fiancé and you're annoyed. Or maybe somebody else got promoted at work and you didn't even get a salary increase. Maybe you can recall some other triggering event.

You're pushing your trolley down the biscuit aisle. Mmmm, what are your favourite biscuits? What are you going to put into your trolley? How many packets are going to satisfy the craving inside you? Maybe those chocolate digestives and the shortbread.

Or maybe your favourite thing is crisps? You reach the sweets and crisps aisle. Which are your favourite flavours: Cheese and onion? Salt and vinegar? Or perhaps you'd like two flavours? That's right: grab the two biggest bags you can find. What else would you put in your trolley to fill up that hole inside? Chocolate? What type? Dark or milk? With nuts? Perhaps with nuts and raisins? Be specific – see yourself adding these to your trolley. Which other sweets will help satisfy your craving?

What about those cream éclairs? They have fresh cream so they must be healthy, right? Or that fizzy drink you haven't tasted for months? Grab a two-litre bottle, put it in your trolley. What about

ice cream? Creamy, cold, mouth-numbing ice cream. Is chocolate your favourite flavour or would you prefer to get stuck into vanilla?

And now you're standing in the queue to pay. What's going to tempt you? A chocolate bar or two? A packet of chocolate-covered toffees or raisins? A selection of delicious dark-chocolate treats? Maybe a packet of crisps to eat on the way home? Go on, load up your trolley.

You're in the car. What are you going to eat on the way home? Better take it out of the shopping bag and have it on the front seat next to you. Now you're eating it while driving. But what will you do with the wrappers? Better hide them so no one knows you've been eating in the car.

You get home and put away your groceries. Now it's time for that major binge. Where are you going to do it? Your lounge? Your bedroom? Do you plan to eat everything at once or will you space it out over a few hours?

Mmmm. Finished? How do you feel? Pretty amazing? You probably have a sugar high. Let's wait six minutes – how do you feel now? A little bloated and ill maybe? Or maybe you don't feel anything at all? What about six hours later when you look back at what has happened? Does any of that guilt and shame surface?

What about in six weeks' time when you realise it wasn't a once-off and you've continued to relapse? Do you hate yourself more now?

What about in six months' time when you no longer fit into your favourite pair of jeans and you've regained all the weight you managed to lose?

What about in six years' time when you realise you're once again starting another diet or exercise programme?

You can stop this movie at any point. Focus on the benefits of the LCHF lifestyle and the long-term satisfaction it brings instead of the short-term 'gain'. Recovery is about progress and not perfection. So take it easy, you're on a journey.

South African life coaching website The Fairy Godmother sums it up perfectly:

'When you get discouraged ask yourself "What would I be doing right now if I wasn't discouraged?"

Then do that.'

⭐

Tips to deal with a relapse

1 Don't be too hard on yourself. Relapses happen to most of us at some stage in our recovery.

2 Move through the experience. Staying stuck will only lead to prolonged relapse behaviours. Take a walk or run, go to a yoga class. Get rid of that energy.

3 Cut out all sugar or sweetness for the next day or two. Cook yourself a wholesome, nourishing meal containing fat, protein and green veg. Stay away from root or dense veg completely.

4 Drink lots of water and herbal teas.

5 Make a gratitude list that focuses on your successes for the day.

6 Share your relapse story with a friend in recovery. There is a saying: 'Shame dies on exposure'.

Nita's story

For as long as I can remember, weight has been an issue for me. My mother put locks on our food cupboards so we couldn't finish the groceries too quickly. I don't recall a childhood of regular healthy meals. It was pretty much a grab-for-yourself on the run. The easiest was bread and jam or peanut butter. Dinners were always meat, a couple of carbs (rice and potatoes) and a veg (always overcooked). I have been vegetarian since I was three years old.

I was very sporty and in spite of bad food and nutrition I managed to keep myself in shape. But I was always chubbier than everyone else. I recall each year looking at my school photos and thinking 'Next year when we take photos, I will be much thinner and look better'. I was ashamed.

→

During university my weight would yo-yo between extremes. From about the time when I was twenty-two I started dieting. I read every book and joined every club (physical and online) and support programme. I've kept journals all my life. On every single day of every single year, every single entry starts with how I'm feeling about my eating and weight.

I developed a pattern of 'clean slate'. I'll start on Monday . . . the first of the month . . . the start of the new year . . . the day my boyfriend comes home etc. I'd start with great intentions and then, within a day or so, fail. And then hate myself. How come I could be so disciplined and successful in everything I did – and I mean everything – but not this? Food and co-dependency became my drugs of choice.

I reached a point where I wasn't enjoying my running because I was lugging an extra 10kg around with me. I hated myself and knew I had tried everything to deal with my eating issues. At this desperate point I found the HELP Program. I wanted:

- the voices in my head to stop calling me names and telling me I was useless.
- certain foods to stop calling me from the fridge, cupboard or shop down the road.
- to stop constantly thinking about food and what I was or wasn't eating.
- to feel fit, strong and energetic. Not wake up with a hangover, regret and remorse and another day of promising myself this time would be different.

What I've noticed is that my relapse starts early. Sitting in the office, in the middle of the afternoon I think 'I must stop and get some bread and milk on my way home'. Trust me, there's no need for bread and milk. It's my addiction planning a stop at the garage shop. But it's so convincing and so powerful that I've given in to it. It's insanity as I walk around the shop with bread and milk in my basket. And chocolate, sweets, ice cream etc. I even convince myself that if anyone were to notice I'd say the sweeties were for my kids. How sick is that? Other people don't care and I don't have kids. Addiction is very real.

→

CHAPTER TWELVE

Since joining the Sugar Free programme I've experienced periods of peace and freedom. I know what it's like and I want it more often. When I've lost a lot of weight I feel fantastic. I started loving running again. But above all, I'm now aware of what is going on. So when I have tough times, I understand. I know to cut myself some slack, which helps me to get back on the horse again. Joining the programme gave me awareness, tools, a system to follow and, most of all, a group of women who're facing the same challenges every single day. This love, support and understanding is the very best grounding for success.

WEEKLY JOURNAL EXERCISE

Take a few minutes to reflect on your week and this stage of your journey:

1   What were your greatest successes this week?
2   How will you build on your successes?
3   Did you stick to your meal plan?
4   Did you maintain abstinence from sugar and carbs?
5   If not, what triggered you to relapse or slip?
    What have you learnt from this experience?
6   What exercise did you do this week?
7   Are you unhappy about anything that happened this week?
8   Have you been affirming yourself?
9   What will you do differently next week to support your journey in recovery positively?
10 Make a list of ten things you are grateful for.

MEASUREMENT	BEGINNING WEEK ONE	21 DAYS	END OF WEEK EIGHT
Weigh yourself. At the gym, at the doctor or at home.			
Take your waist measurement. This is the narrowest point on your torso.			
Take your hip measurement. Feel for your hipbones and measure across the widest part.			
(If female) Take your bust measurement. Take two measurements: under your bust and across your breasts.			
What are your overall energy levels? Rate out of 10 (0 is no energy and 10 is on top of the world).			
What is your mood generally? Mostly irritable and annoyed? Do you look forward to the day or feel grumpy when you wake up? Reflect on this in your journal.			

Affirmation

I can start
my day over
at any time.
I deserve
recovery.

USEFUL RESOURCES

A Course in Weight Loss: 21 Spiritual Lessons for Surrendering Your Weight Forever by Marianne Williamson (HarperCollins, 2012). If your thinking doesn't change, even if you lose weight you'll retain a subconscious urge to gain it back. It's less important how quickly you lose weight, than how holistically you go about it.

Fat Chance: Beating the Odds Against Sugar, Processed Food, Obesity and Disease by Dr Robert Lustig (Hudson Street Press, 2012). The man who exposed the ugly truth in his lecture Sugar: The Bitter Truth explores and challenges the science and politics that helped create chronic lifestyle disease conditions over the past thirty years.

Breakfast	Lunch	Dinner	Snacks	Drinks
Warm Chia Seed Breakfast Mug (see recipe)	Salad (salad leaves, cucumber, peppers, tomatoes, celery) with any protein option (100–150g) with lemon and olive oil dressing – can also sprinkle some seeds on top	2 eggs scrambled with 50g salmon, 50g shredded spinach, 4 florets of broccoli and 25g butter	**Consume up to 2 snacks per day and only when hungry** 10 olives Up to 30g hard cheese 10 Parmesan Crisps with 1 tbsp homemade Guacamole or homemade salsa ½ an avocado topped with balsamic vinegar 50g nuts (not peanuts) 1 Fat Bomb	6–8 glasses of water Tea and coffee (herbal or decaf if you prefer) In coffee and tea, try sticking with double cream or unsweetened almond or coconut milk

Breakfast	Lunch	Dinner	Snacks	Drinks
2 Egg and Parma Ham Cups (see recipe) served with 1 handful of spinach wilted with 2 tsp butter	Super Green Soup with 1 slice Nut and Seed Loaf (see recipe)	Smoked salmon and cream cheese stir-fry: stir-fry ½ a red pepper. ½ a green pepper, ½ a yellow pepper, asparagus, kale and red onion; stir in 75g smoked salmon and 30g cream cheese and season to taste; top with grated Parmesan cheese (optional)	**Consume up to 2 snacks per day and only when hungry** 10 olives Up to 30g hard cheese 10 Parmesan Crisps with 1 tbsp homemade Guacamole or homemade salsa ½ an avocado topped with balsamic vinegar 50g nuts (not peanuts) 1 Fat Bomb	6–8 glasses of water Tea and coffee (herbal or decaf if you prefer) In coffee and tea, try sticking with double cream or unsweetened almond or coconut milk

Breakfast	Lunch	Dinner	Snacks	Drinks
3 tbsp natural whole-milk yogurt with 50g sugar-free Nut and Granola (see recipe) and 50g berries	Creamy Avocado Soup (see recipe) with 2 seed crackers	Chicken 'fajitas': stir-fry chicken strips (plain) with sliced red onion (¼) and red pepper (½), seasoned with salt, cumin and paprika. Serve in iceberg lettuce leaves, topped with guacamole (1 tbsp) and salsa (1 tbsp)	**Consume up to 2 snacks per day and only when hungry** 10 olives Up to 30g hard cheese 10 Parmesan Crisps with 1 tbsp homemade Guacamole or homemade salsa ½ an avocado topped with balsamic vinegar 50g nuts (not peanuts) 1 Fat Bomb	6–8 glasses of water Tea and coffee (herbal or decaf if you prefer) In coffee and tea, try sticking with double cream or unsweetened almond or coconut milk

DAY 53

Breakfast	Lunch	Dinner	Snacks	Drinks
3 rashers of bacon with 50g cream cheese and 50g berries	1 Mocha Protein or Green Smoothie (see recipes)	Tomato and Prawn 'Pasta' (see recipe)	**Consume up to 2 snacks per day and only when hungry** 10 olives Up to 30g hard cheese 10 Parmesan Crisps with 1 tbsp homemade Guacamole or homemade salsa ½ an avocado topped with balsamic vinegar 50g nuts (not peanuts) 1 Fat Bomb	6–8 glasses of water Tea and coffee (herbal or decaf if you prefer) In coffee and tea, try sticking with double cream or unsweetened almond or coconut milk

DAY 54

Breakfast	Lunch	Dinner	Snacks	Drinks
Egg, salmon and avocado platter: 3 eggs (cooked any way you like), 50g salmon (any kind) ½ an avocado and 6 cherry tomatoes	Steak (100g uncooked weight) and blue cheese salad: (up to 30g cheese), 1 handful of young spinach leaves, 1 handful of rocket, ½ green pepper, 50g cucumber, 3 celery stalks	Crème Fraîche and Coriander Chicken (see recipe) served with a large side salad drizzled with 1 tbsp of olive oil	**Consume up to 2 snacks per day and only when hungry** 10 olives Up to 30g hard cheese 10 Parmesan Crisps with 1 tbsp homemade Guacamole or homemade salsa ½ an avocado topped with balsamic vinegar 50g nuts (not peanuts) 1 Fat Bomb	6–8 glasses of water Tea and coffee (herbal or decaf if you prefer) In coffee and tea, try sticking with double cream or unsweetened almond or coconut milk

DAY 55

Breakfast	Lunch	Dinner	Snacks	Drinks
3 tbsp natural whole-milk yogurt with 50g sugar-free granola with 50g of berries	Warm goat's cheese and walnut salad: 30g goat's cheese, 30g walnuts, 1 handful of young spinach leaves, 1 handful of rocket, ½ green pepper, 50g cucumber, 3 celery stalks	Spanish omelette: 3 eggs mixed with diced 30g chorizo, chopped red pepper (½) and paprika; served topped with cream cheese (30g)	**Consume up to 2 snacks per day and only when hungry** 10 olives Up to 30g hard cheese 10 Parmesan Crisps with 1 tbsp homemade Guacamole or homemade salsa ½ an avocado topped with balsamic vinegar 50g nuts (not peanuts) 1 Fat Bomb	6–8 glasses of water Tea and coffee (herbal or decaf if you prefer) In coffee and tea, try sticking with double cream or unsweetened almond or coconut milk

Breakfast	Lunch	Dinner	Snacks	Drinks
3 eggs scrambled with butter, mixed with ½ an avocado, chopped ½ red pepper and 30g feta cheese	Thai Green Curry (see recipe) with 1–2 seed crackers or 1 slice of Nut and Seed Loaf (see recipe)	Portuguese-Style Piri-Piri Chicken (see recipe) with Cauliflower Rice (see recipe), pancetta, Brussels sprouts and garlic	**Consume up to 2 snacks per day and only when hungry** 10 olives Up to 30g hard cheese 10 Parmesan Crisps with 1 tbsp homemade Guacamole or homemade salsa ½ an avocado topped with balsamic vinegar 50g nuts (not peanuts) 1 Fat Bomb	6–8 glasses of water Tea and coffee (herbal or decaf if you prefer) In coffee and tea, try sticking with double cream or unsweetened almond or coconut milk

Vegetarian Meal Plan Week 4 and 8

Breakfast	Lunch	Dinner	Snacks	Drinks
3 tbsp natural whole-milk (or Greek) yogurt mixed with 50g sugar-free Nut Granola (see recipe) and 50g of berries	Mediterranean vegetables (peppers, aubergine, onions and courgettes) and halloumi skewers served with a large salad dressed with olive oil and balsamic vinegar	2 Spinach and Courgette Burgers (see recipe) topped with Cheddar cheese and served with a large salad drizzled with olive oil	**Consume up to 2 snacks per day and only when hungry** 10 olives Up to 30g hard cheese ½ an avocado topped with balsamic vinegar 50g nuts (not peanuts) 1 Fat Bomb	6–8 glasses of water Tea and coffee (herbal or decaf if you prefer) In coffee and tea, try sticking with double cream or unsweetened almond or coconut milk

DAY 51

Breakfast	Lunch	Dinner	Snacks	Drinks
Egg 'muffins': whisk together 4 eggs, chopped tomato, green pepper and onion. Pour into buttered muffin tins and fill halfway. Bake in the oven at 160°C for 15 minutes or until cooked	Creamy Avocado Soup (see recipe) with 2 slices of Nut and Seed loaf (see recipe)	2 slices of Cauliflower Pizza (see recipe), served with Celeriac Chips (see recipe)	**Consume up to 2 snacks per day and only when hungry** 10 olives Up to 30g hard cheese ½ an avocado topped with balsamic vinegar 50g nuts (not peanuts) 1 Fat Bomb	6–8 glasses of water Tea and coffee (herbal or decaf if you prefer) In coffee and tea, try sticking with double cream or unsweetened almond or coconut milk

DAY 52

Breakfast	Lunch	Dinner	Snacks	Drinks
3 tbsp natural whole-milk (or Greek) yogurt mixed with 1 tbsp double cream (optional), 1 tbsp coconut flakes, 30g mixed nuts and 50g berries	Spring onion scrambled eggs: up to 3 eggs scrambled with coconut milk, mixed with chopped spring onion and sprinkled with fresh dill	Cream cheese and vegetable stir-fry: Stir-fry together 1 handful of spinach, 1 handful of kale, ½ a courgette, ½ a red pepper, ½ a yellow pepper, ½ a green pepper, 2 cloves of garlic and ¼ of an onion. Stir in 50g cream cheese and 50g of mozzarella cheese and top with 30g of walnuts and sunflower seeds	**Consume up to 2 snacks per day and only when hungry** 10 olives Up to 30g hard cheese ½ an avocado topped with balsamic vinegar 50g nuts (not peanuts) 1 Fat Bomb	6–8 glasses of water Tea and coffee (herbal or decaf if you prefer) In coffee and tea, try sticking with double cream or unsweetened almond or coconut milk

DAY 53

Breakfast	Lunch	Dinner	Snacks	Drinks
Warm Chia Seed Breakfast Mug (see recipe)	Green Smoothie (see recipe) with 3 celery stalks and almond butter	Spiced omelette: 3 large eggs whisked with 4 tsp milk or double cream, finely chopped onion and red pepper, coriander, cumin and ½–1 tsp chilli powder. Serve with homemade salsa or guacamole	**Consume up to 2 snacks per day and only when hungry** 10 olives Up to 30g hard cheese ½ an avocado topped with balsamic vinegar 50g nuts (not peanuts) 1 Fat Bomb	6–8 glasses of water Tea and coffee (herbal or decaf if you prefer) In coffee and tea, try sticking with double cream or unsweetened almond or coconut milk

Breakfast	Lunch	Dinner	Snacks	Drinks
Berry Smoothie (see recipe)	Super Green Soup (see recipe) served with 1 slice of Nut and Seed Loaf (see recipe) with butter	Aubergine 'pizzas': cut aubergine into 1cm discs (up to 8 slices), spread with sun-dried tomato paste, top with a slice of mozzarella and a slice of Cheddar cheese and sprinkle with basil. Grill for 5–10 minutes. Serve with sautéed spinach	**Consume up to 2 snacks per day and only when hungry** 10 olives Up to 30g hard cheese ½ an avocado topped with balsamic vinegar 50g nuts (not peanuts) 1 Fat Bomb	6–8 glasses of water Tea and coffee (herbal or decaf if you prefer) In coffee and tea, try sticking with double cream or unsweetened almond or coconut milk

Breakfast	Lunch	Dinner	Snacks	Drinks
Egg and avocado platter: 3 eggs (cooked any way you like) and ½ an avocado, and 6 cherry tomatoes	Caprese salad	Mushroom Stroganoff with Cauliflower Rice (see recipes)	**Consume up to 2 snacks per day and only when hungry** 10 olives Up to 30g hard cheese ½ an avocado topped with balsamic vinegar 50g nuts (not peanuts) 1 Fat Bomb	6–8 glasses of water Tea and coffee (herbal or decaf if you prefer) In coffee and tea, try sticking with double cream or unsweetened almond or coconut milk

Breakfast	Lunch	Dinner	Snacks	Drinks
3 tbsp natural whole-milk (or Greek) yogurt mixed with 1 tbsp double cream (optional), 1 tbsp coconut flakes, 30g mixed nuts and 50g berries	Sugar-free Bruschetta (see recipe)	Sweet Potato Frittata (see recipe)	**Consume up to 2 snacks per day and only when hungry** 10 olives Up to 30g hard cheese ½ an avocado topped with balsamic vinegar 50g nuts (not peanuts) 1 Fat Bomb	6–8 glasses of water Tea and coffee (herbal or decaf if you prefer) In coffee and tea, try sticking with double cream or unsweetened almond or coconut milk

13   What's next?

So you've made it. Eight weeks of Sugar Free. Take some time to congratulate yourself. Let it sink in that you've put in place all the habits and tools to help you continue a life that's sugar- and carb-free.

Of course that doesn't mean it will always be smooth sailing. Do you remember what we said in Chapter Two about being an addict?

Addiction is chronic and progressive. This means the condition never goes away and the symptoms get worse over time if not treated. Recovery from addiction is possible but requires both abstinence from the addictive substance and/or behaviour, and daily maintenance by the addict.

In this chapter we'll help you set up your life so that you can continue to be Sugar Free.

Life after the eight weeks by nutritionist Emily Maguire
In order to really reset your body away from sugar cravings we would advise that you continue to follow the eating plan as set out in this book for at least another eight weeks. This is a new way of life and if you change your diet too soon you run the risk of undoing the good work you have achieved.

As you continue in your Sugar Free lifestyle, there are – in very general terms – two main ways of approaching LCHF.

1
MAINTAINING A DAILY CARBOHYDRATE INTAKE OF 50G OR LESS
If you are still looking to lose weight or body fat, then maintaining a carbohydrate level of 50g or less is advisable. (Once you have achieved your weight-loss goal and maintained it for a minimum of one month you might look at making adjustments.) This level of carbohydrate intake would also be advisable for diabetics and individuals who are insulin resistant or have problems with blood sugar levels. In order to determine this, we would recommend that you have your blood sugar measured regularly throughout the programme. If your levels remain high (or low), then staying at 50g would probably be best for you. You can use a blood glucose checker available from high-street pharmacies or online, or visit your GP/practice nurse. If you are diabetic and/or are on medication, then please do not make any changes to your diet or treatment without first seeking medical advice.

JOURNAL EXERCISE

Let's look at your journey over the past eight weeks:

1   Compare your measurements between Week One and Week Eight (refer back to the Check-in exercise for those weeks).
2   Compare your energy levels between Week One and Week Eight (refer back to the Check-in exercise).
3   Compare your general mood between Week One and Week Eight (refer back to the Check-in exercise).
4   What was your biggest learning curve while doing the programme?
5   Where could you focus more attention?
6   Review your abstinence statement from Week One. Is there anything you should add or change?

Now take a few minutes reviewing your Weekly journals written during the past eight weeks:

1   What were your greatest successes?
2   How will you build on your successes?
3   Did you stick to your meal plans?
4   Did you maintain abstinence from sugar and carbs?
5   If not, what triggered you to relapse or slip? What have you learnt from this?
6   What exercise did you do?
7   Are you unhappy about anything that happened?
8   Have you been affirming yourself?
9   What will you do differently to support your journey in recovery positively?
10   Make a list of all the things you are most grateful for.

Now make a list of things you can do to ensure your future is Sugar Free.

Best for you if:
- you are looking to lose weight
- you have insulin resistance
- you carry most of your weight around your belly

- you have hypo/hyperglycemia (low or high blood sugar)
- you are diabetic

2

MAINTAINING A
CARBOHYDRATE INTAKE OF
50–120G PER DAY

Under normal conditions, consuming 50g of carbs or less is generally considered the sweet spot for getting into a ketogenic range – when your body is using fat (body fat or dietary fat) to provide energy. For many individuals it may not be necessary to follow a ketogenic LCHF approach. Equally, some individuals (mainly active people) can consume more carbohydrates and still be in a ketogenic range. And if you're not hungry it's easier to follow a diet. While the added benefit of satiety from ketosis definitely helps, it is not the only reason why someone will maintain new dietary habits. Social and cultural reasons may come into play, and for some people, increasing the carbohydrates slightly can make sticking with an LCHF lifestyle much more sustainable. To find a

Michele's story

Looking back, weight has been an issue that's defined me as a person for the past thirty to thirty-five years of my life. My earliest memories of bad eating habits date to when I was eight or nine years old. I'd take all my weekly pocket money, go down to the corner shop and spend it all on sweets. I finished eating them before I even got home. Food was my source of comfort from early on.

As I reached my teens, I remember feeling bigger than the other girls at school. I always felt ashamed of my body as I progressed into my adolescent years. From my early teens until the age of twenty I was probably about 10kg overweight. Once I left school I discovered 'fad' diets and attempted to keep my weight in check with, for instance, the grapefruit diet or the cabbage diet. I lost weight but within a short period the original weight plus more would be back. It was never sustainable.

I met my husband in my early twenties. While we were going out I managed to control my weight to an extent but I was at least 10kg overweight. My husband didn't worry about my weight – from the beginning he loved and accepted me for who I was and not for how much I weighed. Within a year of our marriage I gained more weight though, and was probably 15–20kg overweight. It got to the point where I just stopped trying.

→

level that is right for you I would recommend gradually increasing your carbohydrate intake and monitoring your weight, hunger and cravings. This is easier than it sounds, as you simply need to increase your intake by 1 portion of non-starchy vegetables to consume approximately an extra 5g of carbohydrate. If you find an increase in any of these things then you have probably consumed too many carbohydrates for your body and will need to reduce them down again. Never exceed 120g of carbs per day. Your major source of carbohydrates will still be non-starchy vegetables and fruits.

Best for you if:
- you are not overweight
- you are looking for more variety
- you do not have problems with high or low blood sugar
- you are physically active

Below you'll find Michele's story. I hope it will motivate you to continue your own journey.

I weighed more than 102kg when I was pregnant with my first son. I was twenty-six when he was born. Although I lost weight afterwards, I never managed to get below 87kg. Over the years I ballooned up to over 100kg again. I was completely disconnected from myself.

My self-esteem was very low. I always felt like I was being judged according to my size and weight. I saw myself as a failure because of all my failed attempts to control my weight. As the years went by I put myself in a very lonely and isolated place.

I was my heaviest when I was forty-four, weighing 144.6kg. I was wearing size 28 clothing. I knew I had to do something; I could no longer ignore my weight. Over four months I lost 13.6kg by myself. Then, motivated to go on a skiing trip at the end of 2008, I managed to lose 32.5kg over the next eight months. I weighed 98.5kg and went skiing. I loved it and came back determined to lose the remaining 25kg of excess weight.

I never managed to do that. Instead I maintained my weight within a 5–7kg range of 98kg for the next two years, which I viewed as progress. I set goals for myself. In 2009, weighing 101kg, I rode a 100-km race. In 2010, weighing 106kg, I climbed Kilimanjaro. Even after Kilimanjaro – which was life-altering – I started to gain weight again. I was nearing 120kg and knew my weight couldn't go back up to where I'd been before.

→

★

**Tips to help you maintain a
Sugar Free lifestyle**

1

SURROUND YOURSELF
WITH SUPPORT
Find meetings, online forums
or organisations that will
support your Sugar Free lifestyle.
Overeaters Anonymous (oa.org) is
part of the twelve-step fellowship;
there are branches around the
world that will welcome you
with open arms. Also remember
the personal network that you
established in Week One. Remind
those people that you still need
their help and support.

2

FIND NEW HOBBIES
OR INTERESTS
Start exploring new hobbies and
interests that will expand you as a
person. Invest some time and effort
in yourself and your recovery. Sign
up for a sugar-free cooking course,

*Then in August 2012 I injured my left knee badly and discovered I needed
surgery. This was my wake-up call. I realised I only had one pair of knees.
To live an active lifestyle and exercise in years to come, I had to lose weight
to take strain off my knees and give my damaged knee the best chance to
recover properly. I started asking myself some very hard questions about
what purpose this weight served in my life.*

*I started on Karen Thomson's Sugar Free programme in November 2012.
I weighed 116.8kg the day I started with a LCHF eating plan. It took a while
to get used to the fact that I didn't have to eat low-fat products, and was
in fact encouraged to eat fats such as full-cream milk, yogurt and cream.
This required a whole new mindset and it took a while to adjust. I had
thought I would miss the carbohydrates, but found they were quite easy
to do without.*

*From a physical point of view I felt much better. What I found particularly
interesting was how emotional I felt when I reduced my carbohydrates. It
confirmed that I was definitely an emotional eater – over the years I'd used
processed carbohydrates to control and disconnect from my emotions.
The longer I stayed away from my 'trigger' foods the easier it became for
me to eat healthily.*

→

join a running club or learn how to paint. Allow yourself to explore this new way of being.

3
START A DAILY GRATITUDE LIST
List at least one thing a day that you are grateful for, even on those days when you are feeling down. Keep your gratitude list close – in your handbag or in your car. Look at the list and remind yourself how far you have come.

4
WATCH FOR TRIGGERS
In Week One I helped you identify your triggers. Be mindful of your triggers and how to manage them.

5
STAY HEALTHY AND GET ENOUGH REST
We generally feel better after eight hours of sleep. Treat your body, mind, spirit and emotions with respect by getting enough sleep, making time to exercise, being

Week by week I was monitored on the programme, and I lost weight consistently. Once the eight weeks were over I continued eating that way and lost 20kg. Although I'd put myself in a better place to reduce knee strain, from a weight perspective after my knee operation, I still had 25kg to lose.

I made a conscious decision that this time I'd give myself the opportunity to lose the last of my excess kilos. I couldn't remember what I'd looked like at a normal weight. I carried on eating the LCHF way while doing a fitness challenge at the gym and lost more. I never lacked energy even though I was doing a variety of exercises.

The fitness challenge ended in January 2014 and at my final assessment they said I was within the normal limits of all my parameters. For the first time in thirty years I was no longer considered overweight or obese; finally I was at a weight that suited my build and age. I now weigh 73kg. I've lost 43.8kg since starting the LCHF eating plan in November 2012.

Physically I feel fit, strong and energetic and in my best physical shape in twenty-five years. Emotionally I have a far more positive outlook. I feel more positive within myself as well. I'm an emotional eater – I'm aware that I need to stay connected to myself and to know what I'm feeling so that I don't revert to using food to deal with my emotions. It's sometimes not a comfortable place to be but it's a more real place.

mindful and sticking to your Sugar Free meal plans.

6

KEEP JOURNALING

Affirm your feelings and activities with journaling. It will keep you accountable to yourself and provide you with a place to write about your struggles and successes. Find inspiring pictures and quotes that you can insert into your journal to help you on those difficult days.

7

BE REASONABLE

Recovery is a journey, so be reasonable with the expectations you set for yourself. Your small successes will help maintain your recovery. Keep doing the next right thing and you will be astounded with the results.

8

EXERCISE

Keep up your exercise routine. A group or a partner will help you stay committed and motivated. Find an exercise in which you can challenge yourself and your beliefs about your limits.

9

PLAN. PLAN. PLAN AND BE PREPARED

In Week One I listed planning as the most effective tool for your recovery. Plan your meals, your snacks, your exercise and time for yourself. I hope that over the past few weeks you have seen how effective planning can be.

10

MINDFULNESS

I explored the concept of mindfulness in Week Seven when I defined it as simply paying attention to your mind and to the present moment. Remember that you're not trying to change anything through mindfulness. Continue to practise your mindfulness every day. Maybe you are ready to start a meditation practice?

Affirmations

Creating a weekly or daily affirmation is another way to help you embody the positive ideals that you have built up over the past eight weeks.

You have probably heard the sayings 'You are what you think' and 'Words have power'. Affirmations are a way to help you think and speak in a more positive way, in a way that helps you to create a positive self.

An affirmation is simply a short empowering and positive statement in the present tense. The word comes from the Latin *affirmare*, which means 'to make steady, or strengthen'. Affirmations play an important role in breaking the cycle of negative thought and the resultant negative self-perception and negative action. If you are thinking of yourself as a confident and lovable person you are less likely to reach for food or sugar when you are in triggering or upsetting situations.

I strongly suggest that you

create a weekly affirmation that you repeat throughout the week. You can write it on sticky notes and put these in places where you will see them throughout the day: your mirror, your journal, your purse, your fridge or your kettle. Better still, programme it as a recurring reminder on your mobile phone. In fact, any place that will remind you to repeat the statement. When you see the note, repeat the affirmation out loud (if you can) or to yourself at least three times in a strong, confident voice.

By repeating the statement a number of times out loud you are trying to influence your brain in a healthy way, almost like reprogramming it. Affirmations are your way of saying 'I can' to the universe over and over again.

JOURNAL EXERCISE

● Make a list of all the people or books that have inspired you in the past.
● Go back to the Useful resources sections during the eight-week programme – add some of those books or websites to your list.
● Add to the list any activity that keeps you connected to yourself and your soul – gardening, taking a belly-dancing class, knitting or hanging out with your children.

You now have a list of resources to keep you inspired. Tap into it at any time.

Here are some examples of affirmations; find ones that resonate with you:

● I am brimming with energy.
● My body is healthy and my mind is tranquil.
● I possess all the necessary qualities to be successful.
● I am courageous and I stand up for myself.
● I always make healthy food choices.
● I am successful and full of hope.
● I use my talents to make a better life for myself, my family and the whole world.
● My business is thriving and expanding.
● My personal relationships are strong and stable.
● I am happy. (Or, I am joyful.)
● I am confident. (Or replace the word confident with any quality that you are trying to embody.)
● I make the right choices for my recovery.
● I choose friends who will support me.
● I let go of the inner critic in my head.
● I have the strength and wisdom to keep on this journey of recovery.

Finding inspiration
It's important to single out people, books, websites and activities that will keep you inspired to live a Sugar Free life – resources you'll be able to turn to again and again to stay motivated.

These are the people and things that keep me inspired

1 My kids are my grounding force. My two free-spirited boys constantly show me what it means to live in the moment, love deeply and express emotions openly and honestly.

2 My husband Steven taught me to question my self-imposed limitations and to follow my heart. He pushes me outside my comfort zone often; it's hard but it's always worth it.

3 My family has been in the public eye for as long as I can remember. They taught me to dream big. As my grandfather Professor Christiaan Barnard used to say, 'It's not that our aim is too high and we miss it, but that it's too low and we reach it.' My mother Deirdre Barnard chronicled her struggles with weight, fame and family issues in *Fat, Fame And Life With Father* (Double Storey, 2003). My gran Louwtjie Barnard played a pivotal role in raising me. My dad Kobus Visser is my greatest supporter. My brother Tiaan is a superbly inspiring individual in his own right.

4 Cardiologist **Dr Aseem Malhotra** who has dedicated his life to improving the health of others. He is fearless, tenacious and brilliant. I am very grateful for his support and encouragement. doctoraseem.com

5 My amazing agent **Gary Wright** who made this book possible. Your dedication, support, encouragement and belief in me go way beyond the call of duty. You truly rock!

6 Adam Pike and his team at **Pike Law** for always keeping me super safe and protected.

7 The Sugar Free/Low Carb community of people I am now blessed to call my friends: Emily Maguire, Christine and Randall Cronau, Zoë and Andy Harcombe, Dr Jeffry Gerber, Dr Jay Wortman, Ivor Cummins, Donal 'o Neill, Dr Jason Fung, Sam Feltham, Yael and Glen Finkel. I absolutely adore you all.

8 Dr Andreas Eenfeldt for being an absolute pioneer in the LCHF movement. Your passion and dedication are amazing. dietdoctor.com

9 Science and health journalist **Gary Taubes** took the time to chat about my 'hare-brained' sugar-addiction treatment idea back in 2011. His groundbreaking books include *Good Calories, Bad Calories* (Knopf Publishing Group, 2007) and *Why We Get Fat: And What To Do About It* (Knopf Publishing Group, 2010). I stay updated about his work at the Nutrition Science Initiative at nusi.org.

10 Michael and **Mary Dan Eades** whom I admire and want to be like. Thank you for opening your hearts to me.

11 Dr Steve Phinney and **Dr Jeff Volek**. Their books *The Art and Science of Low Carbohydrate Living* (Beyond Obesity LLC, 2011) and *The Art and Science of Low Carbohydrate Performance* (Beyond Obesity LLC, 2011) are a must if you're interested in this way of living.

12 Dr Eric Westman and **Jimmy Moore** are leaders (and lovely people) in the low-carb shake-up. They co-authored *Cholesterol Clarity: What The HDL Is*

Wrong With My Numbers? (Victory Belt Publishing, 2013) and *Keto Clarity: Your Definitive Guide to the Benefits of a Low-Carb, High-Fat Diet* (Victory Belt Publishing, 2014) to dispel the nutritional myths we've been told.

13 The **amazing women** spreading the low-carb message: Dr Caryn Zinn, Nina Teicholz, Maryanne Demasi, Dr Ann M Childers, Fransizka Spritzler, Cassie Bjork and Libby from Ditch the Carbs. Visit their blogs, read their books and be inspired.

14 Movement. Yoga teaches me to go with the flow. Running helps me to get through emotions, situations and events.

15 The great anti-sugar pioneers: **Dr Robert Lustig**, **David Gillespie**, **Damon Gameau** and **Dr Nicole Avena**. Find them online or on YouTube videos.

16 My friend **Rita Fernandes Venter** has over 150,000 people in her Facebook group Banting 7 Day Meal Plans. Join in and be inspired.

17 My safe space, a little mountain retreat called Tumbela created by my very wise, kind and loving mentor Val Valentini.

18 Professor Tim Noakes, truly a giant among men. Words cannot express my admiration and gratitude for the role he plays in my life.

19 My greatest Sugar Free inspiration comes from every person who completes the Sugar Free Revolution (thesugarfreerevolution.com) and HELP Program (helpdiet.co.za) and continues with their life in recovery. Huge gratitude to Jemima-Faye Goodall, Lisa Sonn, Amy Daniels and Michele Riley for carrying the sugar addiction message wherever they go.

20 Thanks to the lovely Hemsley sisters for leading the real food movement in the UK. www.hemsleyandhemsley.com Also Sjaniël Torrell for being passionate and courageous in her quest for vibrant health. www.chemistryof wellness.com

Remember that your true search is not for weight loss or external beauty but for yourself. It's up to you to decide your own worth and how far you're willing to go to restore yourself emotionally, mentally, physically and spiritually. It doesn't matter how long it takes – what's important is that you take the first steps and keep on the path.

For more inspiration and thoughts see thesugarfreerevolution.com. Please share your journey and passion with me on Facebook, Twitter and Instagram.

14   Recipes

What about experimenting with some recipes?

Do you have a favourite savoury recipe you could adapt to your new LCHF lifestyle? Take a morning off to experiment in your kitchen. We all benefit from inspiration so please share your ideas at thesugarfreerevolution.com. But in the meantime, here are some tempting recipes to add to your repertoire and help you live a sustainable sugar-free life.

Anything else?

Throughout the eight-week programme I've encouraged you to avoid sugar and any natural or artificial sugar substitutes. Yet at some point in the future (it could even be now) you may feel as if your sugar cravings are under control. If you're ready to add a moderate amount of sweetness back into your diet – perhaps a sugar-free dessert at a dinner party – then try the decadent desserts that follow. The great bit is they use no sugar at all. Like all treats, they should be eaten only occasionally.

Warm Chia Seed Breakfast Mug

The chia seeds absorb the liquid to make 'porridge'. This takes at least six hours, so prepare in the mug, leave in the fridge overnight and warm it through in the morning.

SERVES 1

100ml coconut milk

100ml water (or 100ml strong coffee)

¼ tsp ground cinnamon

1 heaped tsp raw cacao powder

2 heaped tbsp chia seeds

- Put the coconut milk and water in a microwaveable mug.
- Stir in the cinnamon and cacao powder.
  When blended, stir in the chia seeds.
- Put the mug in the fridge overnight until the mixture has 'set'.
- To serve, microwave the mixture in the mug for 60 seconds and you'll have ready-to-eat warm porridge. Alternatively, bring some water to a simmer in a large pan. Stand heat-proof mugs containing the chia mixture in the hot water for about 5 minutes to heat the porridge.

Nut Granola

This can be stored in an airtight container for 3 weeks.

MAKES APPROX. 12 X 40G SERVINGS
200g coconut flakes
100g almonds
30g macadamia nuts
40g sunflower seeds
40g pumpkin seeds
20g flaxseeds (linseeds)
20g sesame seeds
2 tsp ground cinnamon
3 tbsp melted coconut oil

- Preheat the oven to 180°C.
- Combine all the ingredients in a bowl and mix well.
- Spread the mixture in a large roasting dish or baking tray (or two medium-sized ones) to ensure the ingredients roast evenly.
- Bake for 20 minutes, shaking the tray every 5 minutes to ensure that the granola doesn't burn.
- Cool and store in an airtight container for up to 3 weeks. Serve with full-fat Greek yogurt.

★

This is really good as it is, but you could make chocolate granola by adding 8 tbsp raw cacao nibs and 8 tbsp raw cacao powder to the mixture once it has cooled.

Berry Smoothie

SERVES 1

75g frozen berries of your choice

60ml cream

60ml coconut cream (remember to shake the tin or carton
   very well before opening)

60ml cold water

2 tsp coconut oil, melted

mint leaves, to serve

- Put the frozen berries, cream, coconut cream,
  water and coconut oil in a bowl.
- Blitz with a stick blender until smooth.
- Pour into a glass and serve garnished with a couple
  of mint leaves.

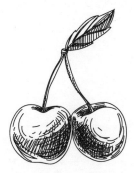

Green Smoothie

SERVES 1

2 large handfuls spinach
¼ large avocado
4 stems broccoli (optional)
1 handful kale
1 slice melon
50g walnuts
100ml coconut milk
2 tbsp full fat Greek yogurt
2 tsp hazelnut butter (or a nut butter of your choice)
100ml unsweetened almond milk
½ scoop (25g) whey protein (optional)
50ml water (optional, depending on how thick you like it)
½ walnut, finely chopped (optional)

- Place all the vegetables, melon and walnuts into a blender and blitz.
- Add the coconut milk, yogurt and nut butter and blitz again.
- Pour in the almond milk and whey protein, if using, and blitz once more.
- If the mixture is still a little thick, add the water.
- Pour into a glass and garnish with chopped walnuts for added crunch, if you like.

Mocha Protein Smoothie

SERVES 1

1 large handful spinach

75g frozen berries

100ml coconut milk

1 tbsp full fat Greek yogurt

1 tsp hazelnut butter (or a nut butter of your choice)

1 scoop of whey protein powder (50g)

1 tbsp coffee granules

½ tbsp cocoa powder

1 tsp stevia or to taste (optional, depending on how
   sweet you like it)

50ml water (optional, depending on how
   thick you like it)

- Place the spinach and berries in a blender and blitz.
- Next, add the coconut milk, yogurt and nut butter and blitz again.
- Pour in the whey protein, coffee, cocoa and stevia and blitz once more.
- If the mixture is a little thick, add the water.
- Pour into a glass to serve.

Egg and Parma Ham Cups

SERVES 1
1 slice Parma ham
1 large egg
1 tsp paprika
1 tsp fresh chives
salt and pepper

- Pre-heat the oven to 180°C.
- Cut the slice of Parma ham in half and use it to line a muffin case, so that the bottom and sides are covered.
- Carefully crack the egg into the Parma ham cup.
- Sprinkle with salt and pepper to taste and bake for around 7–10 minutes, until the egg is cooked through.
- Garnish with paprika and chives, then serve immediately.

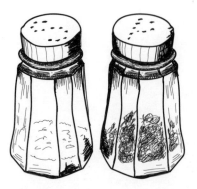

Protein Pancakes

SERVES 1

1 egg
½ scoop (25g) whey protein powder
30g butter at room temperature
1 tsp coconut oil
2 tsp hazelnut butter, for topping (optional)
6 strawberries, hulled and chopped, for topping (optional)

- Whisk the egg and add the protein powder and butter. Mix together until well combined.
- Heat the coconut oil in a frying pan and ladle a spoonful of the mixture into the middle of the hot pan.
- Cook for 2–4 minutes on one side, keeping the pan moving so it does not stick. Turn the pancake over and cook for a further 2–4 minutes, or until golden brown.
- Serve warm with nut butter and strawberries or any other low-sugar fruit. They can also be eaten cold and make an excellent snack.

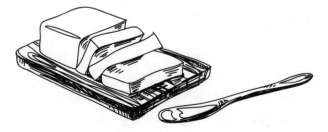

Creamy Avocado Soup

SERVES 2
2 avocados
100ml sour cream
100ml double cream
250ml chicken stock
salt and pepper, for seasoning
1 handful of coriander, to serve

- Slice the avocados, remove the stones and cut up the flesh.
- Blitz the avocado in a food processor with half the quantities of sour cream and double cream.
- Heat the chicken stock in a pan. Once hot add the rest of the sour and double cream and stir gently until mixed.
- Gradually stir the avocado mix into the stock and slowly heat, without bringing it to the boil.
- Season with salt and pepper to taste and serve in a bowl, garnished with sprigs of coriander.

Super Green Soup

SERVES 2 AS A STARTER OR 1 AS A MAIN COURSE

250ml water

3 large handfuls kale

2 handfuls spinach

2 handfuls shredded cabbage

½ trimmed leek

6 florets broccoli

3 baby courgettes or ½ large courgette

2 tbsp coconut oil

1 tsp basil

1 tsp oregano

1 tsp salt

1 tsp pepper

- Place the water in a large saucepan and bring to the boil.
- Add all the vegetables and boil for 10–15 minutes, until all the vegetables are soft.
- Transfer into a food processor or use a hand blender and blitz the vegetables together to form a smooth consistency.
- Stir in the coconut oil, herbs, salt and pepper and blitz again.
- Serve immediately or store in the fridge until required. This can also be stored in the freezer and defrosted when needed.

Caprese Salad

SERVES 1
100g mozzarella
2 large tomatoes
7–8 basil leaves
1–2tsp salt
3 tbsp olive oil

- Slice the mozzarella and tomato into 1cm thick rounds.
- On a large plate, arrange a slice of mozzarella, tomato and a basil leaf and repeat in this pattern until all the ingredients are used up.
- Season with salt (and pepper if desired) and drizzle with a generous amount of olive oil.

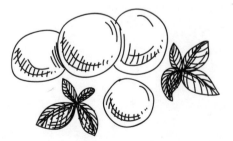

CHAPTER FOURTEEN

Salad Niçoise

SERVES 4

For the French vinaigrette
(Makes about 1½ cups, which can be stored in a
glass container for approximately 3 weeks)
240ml extra virgin olive oil
120ml apple cider vinegar
2 tsp Dijon mustard
1 large garlic clove, crushed
¼ tsp mustard powder
salt and freshly ground black pepper, to taste

For the salad
250g blanched green beans
3 x 120g tins tuna (preferably in water or brine), drained
4 large hard-boiled eggs, sliced
2 medium ripe tomatoes, quartered
85g (approx 3 handfuls) salad greens

- For the dressing, combine the oil, vinegar,
  Dijon mustard and garlic in a blender or small food
  processor and blend until the dressing is thick and
  creamy (emulsified).
- Whisk in the mustard powder and a generous amount
  of salt and pepper. Taste and adjust the seasoning
  if necessary, to taste.
- This dressing will make more than you need for
  one salad; the remaining vinaigrette can be refrigerated
  for a few weeks.
- For the salad, combine all the ingredients in a bowl and
  drizzle with the dressing. Serve with a generous
  grinding of freshly ground black pepper.

Sugar-free Bruschetta

SERVES 1

2 ripe plum tomatoes

1 clove garlic

1 tbsp olive oil

1 tbsp balsamic vinegar

6 fresh basil leaves

1 tsp salt

olive oil, to dress

Seed Crackers (page 215) or slice of
   Nut and Seed Loaf (page 214)

- Peel and dice the tomatoes into small chunks.
- Chop the garlic and mix with the tomato.
  Add the olive oil and vinegar and mix well.
- Stir in the basil leaves and allow the mixture to sit in
  the fridge for one hour.
- Serve on top of seed crackers or a toasted slice of
  Nut and Seed Loaf and drizzle with olive oil.

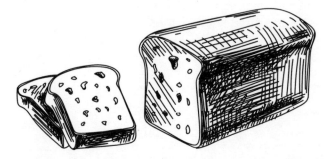

Coconut Camembert with Berry Salad

SERVES 2

½ Camembert cheese, cut into 4 wedges

1 egg, beaten

2 tbsp fine desiccated coconut, for coating

olive oil for frying

30g baby spinach

5 cherry or baby plum tomatoes

10 slices cucumber

40g berries of your choice

balsamic vinegar, to serve

- Cut half a Camembert cheese into 3 equal wedges.
- Dip each wedge of Camembert in the beaten egg and then into the coconut to coat it all over.
- Put the olive oil in a small pan and heat on medium.
- Add the Camembert wedges to the hot oil and cook for 30 seconds to 1 minute on each side. The coating should be golden brown when ready.
- Make a salad by tossing together the spinach, tomatoes, cucumber slices and berries.
- Serve the Camembert wedges on the salad, drizzled with balsamic vinegar.

Baked Eggs with Mozzarella and Asparagus

SERVES 1

100g asparagus
salt and pepper
2 eggs
50g mozzarella
2 tbsp Parmesan, to serve

- Preheat the oven to 180°C.
- Chop the asparagus into bite-sized pieces then place in a baking tray and season.
- Bake the asparagus for 10 minutes.
- Remove the asparagus from the oven and crack the eggs onto the asparagus, then season again.
- Return the baking tray to the oven for 2–3 minutes then remove and scatter the mozzarella, torn into pieces, on top. Cook for a further 5 minutes.
- Remove from the oven and sprinkled on the Parmesan to serve.

CHAPTER FOURTEEN

Baked Eggs in Tomato Sauce

SERVES 4
4 eggs (depending on size)
50g grated mature Cheddar cheese

Tomato sauce
dash of olive oil
1 red onion, finely sliced
1 garlic clove, chopped
2 x 400g cans chopped tomatoes
pinch of salt
pinch of ground black pepper

- To make the tomato sauce, heat the oil in a saucepan and add the onion, garlic, tomatoes, salt and pepper.
- Bring to the boil, then reduce the heat and simmer until thickened, stirring regularly.
- Preheat the oven grill.
- Pour the tomato sauce into a baking dish and make four wells with the back of a spoon.
- Crack one egg into each well in the tomato sauce and sprinkle with grated cheese.
- Bake for about 10 minutes, until the cheese is bubbling and the eggs have set.
- Serve on a bed of fresh rocket, sprinkled with shredded fresh basil or some crushed, crisply grilled bacon. Serve for breakfast, lunch or dinner.

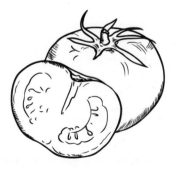

Coconut Chicken

SERVES 1
1 medium chicken breast
1 egg
2 tbsp coconut flour
1 tbsp desiccated coconut

For the salsa
(omit if you are on a strict LCHF/Banting diet)
½ mango
½ red chilli (or a whole one of you prefer your food spicy)
1 clove garlic
juice of 1 lime

- Line a baking tray with foil and preheat the grill to a medium heat (180°C).
- Remove any skin and sinews from the chicken breast and set aside. Whisk the egg in one bowl and in another mix together the coconut flour and desiccated coconut.
- Dip the chicken in the egg mixture and then the coconut flour, turning to make sure that it is completely coated.
- Place the coconut-covered chicken on the baking tray and grill for 20–25 minutes, or until cooked through.
- Whilst the chicken is cooking, make the salsa dressing. Finely dice the mango and chop the garlic and chilli. Mix them all together with the lime juice.
- Place the mango salsa in the fridge until you are ready to serve. Use 2 tbsp to go with this chicken – the salsa makes enough for 4 servings.
- Serve the chicken and salsa with your favourite vegetables. If you are following a slightly higher low-carbohydrate diet, this goes really well with sweet potato fries.

Chicken Parmesan

SERVES 2

For the chicken

2 large eggs

90g grated Parmesan

2 medium chicken breasts

salt and pepper to season

50g mozzarella, grated

For the tomato sauce

½ can (200g) chopped tomatoes

2 tbsp tomato purée

1 tsp basil

1 tsp oregano

½ tsp paprika

1 tsp balsamic vinegar

1 tbsp chopped garlic

- Preheat the oven to 190°C.
- In a wide, shallow bowl crack open the eggs and whisk together
- Put the Parmesan cheese in a similar, separate bowl.
- Dip one of the chicken breasts first into the egg and then into the cheese, turning it each time to ensure that it is properly coated.
- Repeat with the second piece of chicken then place both breasts on a baking tray and cook for 20–25 minutes, until cooked through.
- Whilst the chicken is cooking, make the tomato sauce by combining all the sauce ingredients in a saucepan.
- Cook over a high heat until bubbling, then reduce to a simmer and allow it to reduce slightly.
- Remove the chicken from the oven. Pour a small amount of the sauce into a baking dish, place the chicken on top and cover with the remaining sauce.
- Place the mozzarella over the chicken and bake in the over for a further 5–10 minutes, until the cheese is melted and bubbling.

Chicken Stuffed with Ham and Cheese

SERVES 2

2 skinless chicken breasts
2 slices ham (any type)
3 slices hard cheese (Cheddar, gruyere etc.)
  per chicken breast
1 medium egg, whisked
2 tbsp ground almonds
butter or coconut oil, for frying

- Slice into the long edge of each chicken breast to create
  a pocket and place the ham and cheese inside.
  Re-shape the chicken breasts to enclose the stuffing.
- Place the whisked egg in one bowl and the ground
  almonds in another, then dip each chicken breast into
  first the egg and then the almonds to coat them.
- Place the chicken in a hot pan with some butter or
  coconut oil and fry for 5 minutes on each side.
  Check that the chicken is cooked through
  before serving.

CHAPTER FOURTEEN

Crème Fraîche and Coriander Chicken

SERVES 2

4 boneless chicken thighs
butter or coconut oil, for frying
1 tsp crushed garlic
4 tbsp crème fraîche
2 tbsp double cream
1 tsp Dijon mustard
1 handful fresh coriander
salt and pepper to taste

- Dice the chicken thighs into bite-sized pieces.
- Heat some butter or coconut oil in a large frying pan. Add the chicken and garlic and cook for about 5 minutes, turning occasionally
- Add the crème fraîche, cream and mustard to the pan and stir until it is combined.
- Allow the mixture to bubble for 1–2 minutes then add the coriander and season with salt and pepper to taste.

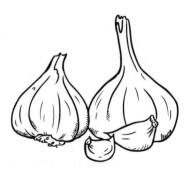

Chicken Aubergine Lasagne

SERVES 4

500g chicken thigh meat
1 tbsp butter or coconut oil
1 onion
3 cloves garlic
400g chopped tomatoes
1 red pepper, chopped
3 tbsp basil
3 tbsp oregano

1 tbsp paprika
2 tbsp tomato purée
salt and pepper
1 large aubergine
180ml double cream
2 tsp mustard
200g grated Cheddar
400g mozzarella

- Dice the chicken and set aside and preheat the oven to 180ºC.
- Heat a large frying pan with 1 tablespoon of butter or coconut oil. Chop the onion and garlic and fry in the oil until the onion is soft.
- Add the chicken to the pan and cook until it is brown.
- In a separate pan, heat the tomatoes, chopped pepper, herbs, tomato purée and salt and pepper to taste. Stir until the mixture is bubbling, then pour over the chicken.
- Mix all the ingredients together and then tip into a large baking dish.
- Slice the aubergine into 1cm thick discs and place on a baking sheet in the oven for 5 minutes.
- To make cheese sauce, pour the cream into a saucepan and heat. Add the mustard and 150g of the grated Cheddar cheese with salt and pepper and stir well until it begins to thicken slightly.
- Next, lay the heated aubergine slices over the chicken and tomato base so that it is fully covered.
- Pour the cheese sauce over the aubergine slices and place in the oven for 15 minutes, then remove and top with the mozzarella, sliced or torn into pieces, and the remaining grated Cheddar. Return the dish to the oven for another 10 minutes or until the cheese has melted and is golden.
- Serve immediately.

Vegetarian Thai Green Curry

We recommend you serve this with cauli-rice, which pushes your veg count up slightly. If you decide instead to serve it on cauli-mash (made with butter, salt and pepper) remember to count 1 fat portion per 1 tsp butter.

SERVES 2
2 tbsp coconut oil
½ onion, diced
1 courgette, diced
3 garlic cloves, chopped
50g white cabbage, shredded
150g frozen peas (thawed)
2 good handfuls of broccoli,
   spinach, mushrooms or
   other light vegetables

Sauce
2 small red onions, roughly chopped
1 tsp green curry paste
1 tbsp grated ginger
8 tbsp coriander leaves,
   plus extra to serve
8 tbsp torn basil leaves
240ml coconut milk
1 tbsp soy sauce
juice of 1 lime or ½ lemon

- In a large saucepan, heat the coconut oil. Sauté the onion, courgette and garlic for about 5 minutes until softened. Set the vegetables aside.
- Make the sauce by placing all the ingredients in a food processor. Blend until smooth.
- Transfer the sauce to the saucepan of cooked veggies. Simmer on low.
- Add the cabbage, peas and other veggies of your choice. Heat through.
- Serve the warm curry with fresh coriander leaves. It's delicious on a bed of steamed cauli-rice. Refrigerate any leftovers in a sealed container for up to three days.

Thai Green Curry

SERVES 2

3 cloves garlic, sliced

½ onion, diced

2 tbsp coconut oil

2 chicken breasts or 4 chicken thighs, cut into thin strips

170g cabbage

1 large handful broccoli, spinach, chopped courgette
  or a combination of green vegetables

For the sauce

240ml coconut milk

120ml chicken stock

small bunch coriander leaves, stalks removed

2 small red onions

small bunch basil leaves, torn

1 tbsp soy sauce

1 tbsp grated ginger

1 tsp green curry paste

1 lime or ½ lemon, juiced

- In a large saucepan, fry the garlic and onion in the coconut oil until golden.
- Add the chicken and fry until cooked through. Set aside while you make the sauce.
- Put all the ingredients for the sauce into a food processor and blend until smooth.
- Transfer the sauce to the pan with the chicken and simmer over a low heat for 10 minutes.
- Add the cabbage and green vegetables and cook for another 5 minutes.
- Serve warm, garnished with fresh coriander. This dish will keep in a sealed container in the fridge for up to three days.

Portuguese-Style Piri-Piri Chicken

SERVES 1

½ lemon, juiced
2 cloves garlic, chopped
2 tsp chopped chilli
1 tsp paprika
1 tsp oregano
60ml apple cider vinegar
1 chicken fillet (or 2 drumsticks)
½ lime, juiced

- Mix all the ingredients together apart from the chicken and lime juice.
- Place the chicken in the mixture, make sure it is well coated and marinate in the fridge overnight.
- When ready, grill the chicken for 25–30 minutes turning occasionally to ensure that it is cooked on both sides and all the way through.
- Once cooked, season with the lime juice and serve with cauliflower rice.

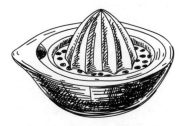

Chicken Tikka Strips

SERVES 1
3 tbsp full fat yogurt
1 tsp paprika
1 tsp chilli powder
1 tsp cumin powder
1 tsp coriander
1 tsp turmeric
1 tsp garam masala
200g mini chicken fillets

- Preheat grill to 180°C.
- In a small bowl combine the yogurt with all the spices and mix thoroughly.
- Next, take each chicken strip and coat it in the mixture so they are all well covered.
- Lay the chicken strips on a foil-lined baking tray. Place under grill and grill for 10–15 minutes, turning occasionally.
- Make sure the chicken is cooked through before removing from the grill. Serve immediately as a hot meal or snack, or allow them to cool and store in the fridge to have as a snack or as part of a salad.

Stuffed Goat's Cheese Turkey Burgers

MAKES 4 BURGERS

200g turkey mince (thigh or breast)
1 tbsp dried basil
1 tbsp dried oregano
1 large egg
3 shallots, finely chopped
1 clove garlic, minced
1 whole chilli or 1 tsp dried chilli (optional)
salt and pepper, to taste.
50g soft goat's cheese
coconut oil, for frying

- In a large bowl, combine the turkey with the herbs. Crack the egg into the mix and, using your hands, start to mix it together.
- Add the shallots, garlic and chilli, then season with salt and pepper and continue to mix until all the ingredients are well combined.
- Take a small handful of the mixture and mould it into a flat patty shape. Place it on a clean plate and add a small piece of goat's cheese to the centre of the burger.
- Make another small burger patty and place it over the one with the goat's cheese in the centre.
- Use your hands to mould the two together so that the burger is sealed and has a smooth edge all the way round.
- Repeat the process with the rest of the mixture to make 4 medium-sized burgers.
- Heat a frying pan with a little coconut oil and fry each of the burgers in turn, flipping to avoid burning.
- Serve topped with grated Cheddar cheese, if you like, and a large side salad. As an optional extra you can add sour cream or homemade salsa.

Bobotie and Coleslaw

Bobotie is a traditional South African dish of spiced minced meat baked with a creamy egg topping. Many cooks have a favourite family recipe: this is a low-carb version.

SERVES 6

3 tbsp butter

1–2 garlic cloves, crushed

2 onions, chopped

500g beef mince (or soya mince)

1 tbsp medium curry powder

1 tsp ground coriander

½ tsp ground ginger

1 tsp ground turmeric

½ tsp ground cinnamon

1 tbsp dried mixed herbs

2 small–medium carrots, grated

2 bay leaves

ground salt crystals or flaked salt
  and ground black pepper

Topping

2 eggs

240ml buttermilk

½ tsp ground salt crystals
  or flaked salt

ground black pepper

Coleslaw

2 carrots, grated

½ white cabbage, finely shredded

120ml sour cream

120ml mayonnaise

1 tsp caraway seeds

ground salt crystals or flaked salt
  and ground black pepper

- Preheat the oven to 190°C.
- Melt the butter in a saucepan and fry the garlic and onions until softened.
  Add the mince and cook, stirring, until it's loose and crumbly.
  Add the spices, herbs, carrots and a bay leaf. Cook for a few more minutes.
  Add salt and pepper to taste.
- Remove the bay leaf and spread the mixture in an ovenproof dish.
- Make the topping by whisking the eggs and then mixing with the buttermilk, salt and pepper. Pour the topping over the mince.
  Place the remaining bay leaf on top and bake, uncovered, for 35 minutes.
- Make the coleslaw by combining all the ingredients;
  serve with the bobotie.

Chilli Con Carne

SERVES 4

4 shallots
2 cloves garlic
butter or coconut oil, for frying
1 red pepper, diced
1 tsp chilli powder
1 tsp paprika
1 tsp cumin
½ tsp oregano
½ tsp cinnamon

400g beef mince
1 x 400g tin chopped
   tomatoes
1 beef stock cube
200ml boiling water
2 tbsp sundried tomato paste
1 x 400g tin kidney beans
grated cheese (optional)
sour cream and guacamole,
   for topping (optional)

- Finely slice the shallots and garlic and fry in a pan over a medium heat with some butter or coconut oil for 5 minutes.
- Add the chopped red pepper, chilli powder, paprika, cumin, oregano and cinnamon, mix well and allow to cook for another 2 minutes, stirring occasionally to avoid sticking.
- Next, add the mince and cook until there are no pink bits left.
- Once the mince is browned, pour in the tinned tomatoes. Dissolve the stock cube in the boiling water and add to the pan with the sundried tomato paste.
- Bring the mixture to a simmer and cook for 10 minutes.
- Drain and rinse the kidney beans, then add them to the frying pan. Bring the pan back to the boil and allow to gently bubble for a final 10 minutes.
- Season with salt and pepper as required and serve immediately with some grated cheese, sour cream and guacamole on top. Additionally, you can also serve it with some seasoned cauliflower rice (see page 221).

Lamb Koftas

MAKES 8 KOFTAS
400g lamb mince
1 onion
3 cloves garlic
1 tbsp ground coriander
1 tbsp ground cumin
½ red chilli
1½ tbsp fresh coriander
1½ tbsp fresh oregano
salt and pepper to season
coconut oil or butter, for frying

- Combine all the ingredients in a large bowl and mix well. Season the mixture with salt and pepper to taste.
- Mould the mixture into 8 equal balls and thread each one onto a wooden skewer (soak these first to prevent the wood from chipping or from burning as you cook).
- Make the koftas into long oval shapes by using your hands to spread the mixture along the skewers.
- Fry the koftas in a large frying pan in a little coconut oil or butter for around 4 minutes each side, or until they are browned and cooked through.

Philly Cheese Steak Stuffed Mushrooms

SERVES 1

2 large flat mushrooms
coconut oil or butter
½ red pepper
½ yellow pepper
½ green pepper
1 shallot
100g strip steak (or any type of steak)
1 tsp sea salt
50g (3 tbsp) full fat cream cheese
½ tsp ground black pepper

- Place the mushrooms on a baking tray, brush with
  1 tbsp of coconut oil or butter and grill for 10 minutes.
  Once golden brown remove from the grill
  and set aside.
- Slice the peppers and shallots and fry in a little
  coconut oil or butter until they are soft.
- In a separate pan, fry the steak with some coconut oil
  or butter until it is cooked to your preference.
- Mix the steak and pepper mix together. Stir in the
  cream cheese and season with the black pepper.
- Spoon the mixture over the grilled mushrooms.

Pork Stroganoff

SERVES 4
1 onion
3 cloves garlic
1 tbsp coconut oil, for frying
450g pork fillet, sliced into thin strips
250g closed cup mushrooms, sliced
200ml double cream
2 tbsp crème fraîche
1 tbsp mustard
1 tsp sundried tomato paste
1 tbsp paprika
1 tsp chilli powder (or to taste)
1 tsp lemon juice (or to taste)
salt and pepper

- Dice the onion and chop the garlic then fry in the coconut oil over a medium heat until the onion is soft.
- Add the pork to the pan and cook until it is brown then add the mushrooms and cook until they are soft.
- Once all is cooked through, pour in the double cream and crème fraîche and mix until all the ingredients are covered. Add the mustard and sundried tomato paste and combine well.
- Lastly, add the paprika and the chilli powder and season with the lemon juice, salt and pepper to taste. You can omit the chilli powder or reduce the quantity if you prefer a less spicy dish.

Mini Salami 'Pizzas'

Mozzarella and Cheddar are classic pizza-topping cheeses, but try these with goat's cheese or halloumi, too.

SERVES 2 (3 PER SERVING)
6 slices salami
2 tbsp sundried tomato paste
50g mozzarella, sliced
30g Cheddar cheese, grated
Dried herbs of your choice: basil, thyme, sage, rosemary

- Preheat the grill to medium.
- Lay the salami slices on a baking tray and spread an even amount of sundried tomato paste on each one.
- Next, layer on a slice of mozzarella and then a layer of Cheddar cheese.
- Sprinkle over your choice of herbs and season with salt and pepper if desired.
- Place the 'pizzas' under the grill for around 5–7 minutes. Do keep an eye on these as they can cook pretty quickly and may be prone to burning.

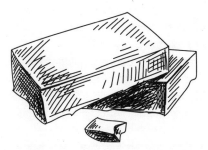

Cauliflower Pizza

SERVES 2

1 small cauliflower, broken into florets

30g Parmesan cheese, grated

30g mozzarella cheese, grated

½ tsp dried oregano

½ tsp dried basil

½ tsp garlic powder

¼ tsp dried chilli flakes

¼ tsp salt

1 egg

For the toppings

4 tbsp homemade tomato sauce (see page 187)

60g mozzarella cheese, grated

toppings of your choice, such as sliced mushrooms,
   peppers or onions, or even an egg

- Preheat the oven to 200°C. Line two baking sheet with non-stick baking paper (or use a silicone baking sheet).
- Place the cauliflower florets in a food processor or blender and pulse until finely chopped.
- Put the cauliflower into a microwave-safe bowl and microwave on High (800 watt; 100%) for 4 minutes. Leave to cool.
- Turn out the cauliflower onto a clean tea towel and, once it is cool enough to handle, wring it tightly. You need to get as much moisture out as possible.
- Place the cauliflower pulp in a mixing bowl and add the cheeses, herbs, spices and the egg. Mix until well combined.
- Form half the mixture into a ball and place it on a baking sheet, then flatten it out using your hands or the back of a spoon into a round about 30cm in diameter. Repeat for the other pizza base.
- Bake for 10–15 minutes until the dough is golden brown, then carefully remove the bases from the oven.
- Preheat the grill. Add your toppings and place the pizzas one at a time under the grill until the cheese has melted.

Sweet Potato Frittata

SERVES 1

½ large sweet potato
coconut oil, for frying
1 shallot, sliced
2 eggs
2 tomatoes
1 tsp basil
1 handful fresh chives
salt and pepper

For the tomato salsa

3 plum tomatoes, diced
1 spring onion, finely sliced
handful of coriander leaves
½ juice of lemon
1 tbsp olive oil
salt and pepper

- Start by making a salsa to accompany the frittata.
  Finely chop the tomatoes and mix with the other
  ingredients. Set this aside while you cook the frittata.
- Dice the potato into small cubes and fry in a pan with
  a little coconut oil for 4–5 minutes until softened.
  Add the shallot and continue to cook until the shallot
  is also soft.
- In a bowl, lightly beat the eggs along with the
  tomatoes, basil, chives and salt and pepper to taste.
- Pour the egg mixture over the potatoes. Move the eggs
  around the pan to avoid sticking and cook through.
  If your pan is safe to use under the grill, you can finish
  the frittata under a hot grill to help to cook it through.
- Serve with the tomato salsa.

Spinach and Courgette Burgers

SERVES 1
4 large handfuls spinach
1 medium or ½ large courgette
1 large egg
1 clove garlic
½ onion
1 tsp basil
1 tbsp ground almonds

- Blitz all ingredients together in a food processor apart from the almonds
- Once combined, gradually add the almonds until the texture has dried slightly.
- Form the mixture into patty shapes, place on a baking tray and grill for 15–20 minutes or until the burgers are golden.

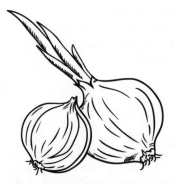

CHAPTER FOURTEEN

Tomato and Prawn 'Pasta'

SERVES 1

100g courgettes (or 3 baby courgettes)

½ onion

1 clove garlic

coconut oil or butter, for frying

80g mushrooms

½ red pepper

100g chopped tomatoes

1 tsp tomato purée

1 tbsp capers

½ tsp mustard

½ tsp garlic salt

75–100g prawns

- Thinly slice the courgette into ribbons. You can do this freehand with a knife or use a peeler or spiraliser. Set the courgette to one side while you prepare the sauce.
- Dice the onion and chop the garlic and fry them in a pan with a little coconut oil or butter.
- Next, finely chop the mushrooms and red pepper add them to the pan with the onion and garlic.
  Continue to fry until the mushrooms are soft.
- Add the chopped tomatoes to the mushroom mixture together with the tomato purée, capers, mustard and garlic salt.
- Remove the sauce from the heat and, with a blender or food processor, blitz until it is smooth and thick.
- Bring a pan of water to the boil and lightly blanch the courgette ribbons for 2–3 minutes while you return the sauce to the heat to warm through.
- Drain the courgette ribbons then pour the sauce over them and top with the prawns. Grill or fry the prawns first if you prefer them hot.

Creamy Mushroom and Ham 'Pasta'

SERVES 1

100g courgettes (3 baby courgettes)

½ onion

1 clove garlic

coconut oil or butter, for frying

80g mushrooms

25ml double cream

25ml coconut milk

1 tsp mustard

½ tsp garlic salt and pepper, to taste

75g ham, finely sliced

grated cheese or finely chopped tomato, to garnish

- Thinly slice the courgettes into ribbon like strips, either freehand with a knife or by using a peeler or spiraliser.
- Place the courgette ribbons in a pan of boiling water and lightly blanch for 2–3 minutes, then plunge into ice-cold water to stop them from cooking further and tip them into a colander to drain.
- Dice the onion and garlic and fry in a little coconut oil or butter until the onion is soft.
- Next, finely chop the mushrooms and add to the onion and garlic, continuing to cook for another 2–3 minutes.
- Pour in the cream and coconut milk. Stir in the mustard and season with the salt and pepper to taste.
- Reduce the pan to a medium heat so it is not boiling. Once the cream has reduced slightly, remove from the heat and tip the creamy sauce into a food processor or, using a hand blender, blitz until it is smooth.
- Heat a little more oil or butter in a frying pan and fry the courgette ribbons with the ham for 2–3 minutes. You can use a combination of different hams, such as Parma and cooked ham, or just choose one type.
- Tip the courgette and ham into a bowl and pour over the sauce. Garnish with some grated cheese or finely chopped tomato for added flavour.

Cheesy Courgette 'Pasta'

SERVES 1

1 large or 2 medium courgettes
coconut oil, for frying
100g full fat cream cheese
2 heaped tbsp crème fraîche
180g grated Parmesan cheese
2 tbsp lemon juice
1 tbsp pumpkin seeds
salt and pepper

- Use a spiraliser or vegetable peeler to make 'noodles' from the courgettes.
- Sauté them in a pan in a little coconut oil for 5 minutes then remove and put to one side.
- Heat up the cream cheese, crème fraîche, Parmesan cheese and lemon juice in a saucepan.
- Add the courgette noodles to the sauce and stir well.
- Season to taste and sprinkle with pumpkin seeds and a little extra Parmesan if desired.

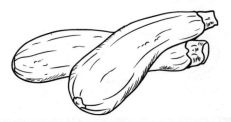

Mushroom Stroganoff

SERVES 2

1 onion

3 cloves garlic

1 tbsp coconut oil, for frying

100g closed-cup mushrooms, sliced

50g shitake mushrooms, sliced

50g oyster mushroom, sliced

150ml double cream

1 tbsp crème fraîche

½ tbsp mustard

1 tsp sundried tomato paste

1 tbsp paprika

1 tsp chilli powder (or to taste)

1 tsp lemon juice (or to taste)

salt and pepper

- Dice the onion and garlic together then fry in the coconut oil over a medium heat until the onion is soft.
- Add the mushrooms to the pan and cook until soft then pour in the double cream and crème fraîche and mix until all the ingredients are covered.
- Add the mustard and sundried tomato paste and combine well, then add the paprika and chilli powder and season with the lemon juice, salt and pepper to taste.

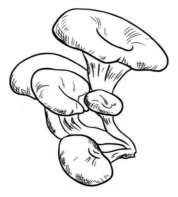

Stuffed Aubergine

SERVES 1

½ aubergine

½ onion, diced

10 cherry tomatoes, diced

½ green pepper, diced

½ red pepper, diced

½ orange pepper, diced

1 tbsp sundried tomato paste

75g mozzarella

50g goat's cheese

- Hollow out the aubergine half. Place the flesh in a frying pan and the skin and outer layer of flesh on a baking tray.
- Grill the hollowed aubergine 'boat' for 10 minutes.
- In a large frying pan, fry the aubergine flesh with the onion, tomatoes and peppers until they are soft. Mix in the sundried tomato paste.
- Place the aubergine mixture into the hollowed out shell. Top with the cheese, torn or crumbled into pieces, and grill until golden.

Cauliflower Mac 'n' Cheese Bake

SERVES 2

butter, for greasing

1 large head cauliflower, cut into small florets

1 tsp salt

250ml cream

60ml cream cheese, cut up into smaller pieces

1 tsp Dijon mustard

180g grated Cheddar cheese. 120g included in recipe,
   60g as topping for bake.

pinch of garlic powder

salt and pepper, to taste

- Preheat the oven to 180°C and grease a 20cm square
  ovenproof dish with butter and set aside.
- Bring a pot of salted water to the boil then cook the
  cauliflower in the boiling water until crisp-tender.
  This should take approximately 5 minutes. Drain well
  and pat between several layers of paper towels to dry.
- Transfer the cauliflower to the baking dish and
  set aside.
- Bring the cream to a simmer in a small saucepan. Add
  the cream cheese and mustard and whisk until smooth.
- Stir in 120g of the grated cheese and allow to melt.
  Season with salt, pepper and garlic.
- Pour the cheese sauce over the cauliflower, top with
  the remaining grated cheese and bake for about
  15 minutes, until browned and bubbling.

Cauliflower Mushroom Risotto

SERVES 2

200g mushrooms

coconut oil or butter, for frying

4 shallots

2 cloves of garlic

1 cauliflower

250ml vegetable stock

200ml double cream

salt and pepper, to taste

fresh thyme, to serve

- Chop the mushrooms and fry in the coconut oil or butter.
- Chop the shallots and garlic and add to the frying pan with the mushrooms.
- Remove any leaves and the tough central stalk from the cauliflower, then grate or blitz the head in a food processor.
- Add the cauliflower to the pan and fry for 2–3 minutes.
- Pour in the stock and bring to boiling point, then reduce the heat to a simmer and add the cream.
- Stir together until the cauliflower is soft and most of the liquid is gone. Season with salt and pepper to taste.
- Remove from the heat and garnish with thyme to serve.

Cauliflower Rice with Pancetta, Brussels Sprouts and Garlic

SERVES 2

1 tsp olive oil or coconut oil
2 cloves of garlic, crushed
65g diced pancetta
10 Brussels sprouts, finely chopped
200g cauliflower rice (see page 213)
10g butter
salt and pepper, to taste

- Heat the oil in a large non-stick frying pan or wok.
  Fry the garlic together with the pancetta.
- Add the Brussels sprouts and mix well
- Add the cauliflower rice and stir-fry for 4–5 minutes
  over medium-high heat.
- Stir in the butter and season with salt and pepper
  to taste.
- Serve as an accompaniment to a main meal.

Cauliflower Rice

SERVES 1
100g cauliflower florets
salt and pepper, to taste
1 tbsp butter

- Grate the cauliflower into a bowl or blitz in a food processor until reduced to rice-like crumbs, and season with salt and pepper.
- Add the butter and cook on high (800 watts; 100%) power in the microwave for 2 minutes. Stand for 2 minutes before serving.
- Alternatively, steam until tender.

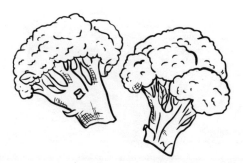

Nut and Seed Loaf

MAKES 1 LOAF (APPROXIMATELY 12 SLICES)

200g mixed seeds

400g nuts of your choice, such as almonds, walnuts,
Brazil nuts, macadamia nuts

3 eggs

4 egg whites

pinch of ground crystals or flaked salt

75g coconut oil, melted, plus extra for greasing

- Preheat the oven to 160 °C and grease a small loaf tin.
- Grind all the seeds and half the nuts in a food
  processor until flour-like in texture. Chop the
  remaining nuts roughly.
- In a separate bowl whisk together the eggs and
  egg whites.
- Combine all the ingredients and mix well.
- Pour the mixture into the loaf tin and bake for
  50–60 minutes.
- Remove from the oven and allow to cool.
  Store in an airtight container for up to four days or
  slice and freeze.

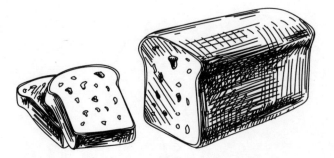

Seed Crackers

Make sure you count the extra protein, fat or veg portions for any toppings used.

Seeds are quite high in carbohydrates, so don't eat too many crackers in one go.
The crackers can be stored for approximately one week in an airtight container.

MAKES 32 CRACKERS
2 tbsp psyllium husks
2 tbsp chia seeds
500ml water
600g seeds of your choice, such as sunflower, sesame, flaxseeds (linseeds
2 tsp ground salt crystals or flaked salt
3 tbsp melted coconut oil

- Mix the psyllium husks, chia seeds and water. Set aside for 5 minutes until it forms a gel-like consistency.
- Add all the seeds, salt and oil to the mixture and combine the ingredients thoroughly. Set aside for 1 hour.
- Preheat the oven to 175°C.
- Line two medium-sized baking trays with silicone sheets or non-stick baking paper. Spread the mixture thinly over the trays.
- Bake for approximately 60 minutes or until the crackers are crisp.
- Remove from the oven, peel off the baking paper and cool. Store in an airtight container.

Celeriac Chips

SERVES 10 (1 SERVING = 90G)
1 whole celeriac
1 tbsp coconut oil, melted
1 tsp dried basil
1 tsp dried oregano
salt and pepper, to taste

- Preheat the oven to 200ºC.
- Peel and slice the celeriac into chip-sized pieces (roughly the size of your thumb).
- Place in a pan of boiling water and blanch for 2 minutes.
- Drain and dry off any excess moisture from the celeriac using kitchen towel, then place in a baking tray.
- Drizzle over the coconut oil and season with the herbs, salt and pepper.
- Bake in the oven for 25–30 minutes, or until golden and cooked through.

Parmesan Crisps

50g Parmesan cheese, grated
paprika, cayenne pepper, salt or garlic granules,
  for seasoning

- Preheat the grill to a medium–low setting and line a baking tray with foil.
- Take small handfuls of the cheese and arrange into small 'crisp' shapes on the baking tray.
  Leave some space between for them to spread a little as they melt.
- If you would like to add different flavours to your crisps, sprinkle over the spice of your choice – paprika, cayenne pepper or garlic granules are all good choices.
- Place the crisps under the grill and cook for 5–10 minutes. Keep an eye on these as they can burn quickly.
- Once they have gone golden brown, remove from the grill and allow to cool. Once they have cooled, begin to peel them off the foil. Take care with this, as the crisps will be fragile and can easily break.
- Serve on their own or with a sour-cream based dip.

Guacamole

SERVES 4
1 clove garlic
3 shallots
1 fresh chilli
2 ripe avocados
6 cherry tomatoes
1 bunch of fresh coriander
juice of 1 lime
2 tbsp of olive oil
sea salt and pepper to taste

- Chop the garlic, shallots and chilli together.
- Cut the avocados in half and remove the stones.
  Scoop out the flesh and mash it.
- Add the chilli, shallots and garlic to the avocado.
- Finely chop the tomatoes and add to the mixture.
- Chop the coriander and stir in along with the lime
  juice and olive oil.
- Combine well and season to taste with salt and pepper.
- Cover and store in the fridge for up to 3 days.

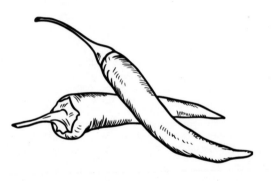

Homemade Sugar-free Mayo

SERVES 4

4 egg yolks at room temperature
1 tbsp apple cider vinegar
1 tsp regular or Dijon mustard
salt and pepper, to taste
165ml olive oil
165ml coconut oil, melted

- Put the egg yolks into a blender or bowl and whisk or blend until smooth.
- Add the apple cider vinegar, mustard and seasoning, and continue to blend until mixed.
- Very slowly add the olive oil while blending or whisking at low speed. Start with a drop at a time until it starts to emulsify, or thicken, and then keep adding slowly until all the oil is incorporated. Repeat with the coconut oil.
- Store in the fridge up to 1 week.

Pesto Sauce

SERVES 1
75g pine nuts
200ml olive oil (leave 50ml aside)
1 large handful fresh basil
50g Parmesan cheese
salt and pepper, to taste
1 tsp lemon juice

- Heat a small saucepan and cook the pine nuts until they are golden. Stir them occasionally to prevent burning.
- Once cooked, place the pine nuts in a food processor with 150ml of the olive oil and all the other ingredients.
- Blitz the ingredients until well mixed, then place in a jar and drizzle over the remaining 50ml olive oil.
- Cover with a lid and keep in the fridge for 10–14 days.

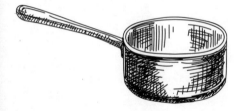

CHAPTER FOURTEEN

Raw Chocolate Ball Pops

Seeds and nuts are quite high in carbohydrates so don't eat too many ball pops at once.

MAKES 8

70g sunflower seeds
120g nuts (almonds, Brazil nuts, macadamias)
2 tbsp chia seeds or flaxseeds (linseeds)
60g almond butter
25g unsweetened desiccated coconut,
    plus extra for rolling
2½ tbsp raw cacao powder
1 tsp ground cinnamon
pinch of sea salt

- Blitz the seeds and nuts in a food processor or blender.
- Transfer to a bowl and add the almond butter, coconut, cacao powder, cinnamon and salt. Combine well.
  Add a drizzle of water only if the mixture is too stiff – the consistency should be firm and hold together nicely.
- Roll into 8 walnut-sized balls. Now roll those balls in the extra coconut. You can also roll in chia seeds (optional).
- Stick in narrow straws to make 'pops'.

Sugar-free Fat Bombs

MAKES 24

30g butter

4 tbsp (60g) extra-virgin, cold pressed coconut oil

2 tablespoon cocoa powder

2 tsp (10g) stevia or 6 drops liquid stevia

2 tbsp double cream

120g nut butter

- In a small saucepan melt the butter and coconut oil together over a low heat.
- Stir in the cocoa powder, stevia, and cream.
  Mix well and continue to heat, but do not let it reach boiling point.
- Carefully spoon half the mixture into small silicone moulds or cupcake trays.
- Spoon 1 tsp of nut butter into the centre of each of the moulds.
- Pour the remaining mixture over the nut butters to cover.
- Place the tray of fat bombs in the freezer for a minimum of two hours. Once fully frozen, remove them from the trays and keep in an airtight container in the freezer.

Nutty Pancakes

Note

If you're eating these with whipped cream and berries, remember to add additional fat and fruit portions.

MAKES 6

100g almond flour

¼ tsp bicarbonate of soda

3 eggs

1 tbsp milk, coconut milk or almond milk

scraped seeds of 1 vanilla pod (optional but delicious)

1 tsp butter or coconut oil

- Put the nut flour and bicarbonate of soda into a mixing bowl. Whisk the eggs together, then gradually stir into the dry ingredients. Once the egg and flour are combined, add the milk (and vanilla, if using) and mix through. Let the batter stand for 5 minutes.
- Heat a small frying pan and melt the butter or coconut oil.
- Add a ladleful of the batter. Cook over medium heat for a few minutes, until bubbles appear on top, then flip the pancake with a spatula and cook the other side.
- Remove from the pan and keep warm while you make the remaining pancakes.
- Serve with whipped cream and fresh or stewed berries.

★

Make your own nut flour by blending nuts such as almonds, walnuts or macadamias in a food processor until they resemble coarse flour. Don't overdo it or your nut flour will turn into nut butter.

Portuguese Custard Tarts

MAKES 10 SMALL TARTS

8 eggs

800ml cream

2 tsp psyllium husks

2 pinches of salt

2 tsp vanilla essence

50ml melted butter, plus extra for greasing

2 tbsp unsweetened desiccated coconut
   (optional)

To serve

cream

ground cinnamon

- Preheat the oven to 220°C. Grease 10 holes of a muffin tin.
- Mix all the ingredients apart from the melted butter in
  a food processor.
- Add the melted butter and mix well.
  You can add desiccated coconut to the mixture (optional).
- Pour the batter into the muffin tin and bake for
  20–30 minutes.
- Serve with 1 tbsp cream and a sprinkle of cinnamon.

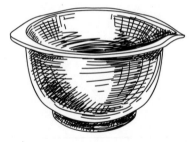

Conversion Tables

OVEN TEMPERATURES

°C	Fan °C	°F	Gas	Description
110	90	225	¼	Very cool
120	100	250	½	Very cool
140	120	275	1	Cool
150	130	300	2	Cool
160	140	325	3	Warm
180	160	350	4	Moderate
190	170	375	5	Moderately hot
200	180	400	6	Fairly hot
220	200	425	7	Hot
230	210	450	8	Very hot
240	220	475	8	Very hot

WEIGHTS FOR DRY INGREDIENTS

Metric	Imperial	Metric	Imperial
7g	¼ oz	400g	14oz
15g	½ oz	425g	15oz
20g	¾ oz	450g	1lb
25g	1 oz	500g	1lb 2oz
40g	1 oz	550g	1¼lb
50g	2oz	600g	1lb 5oz
60g	2 oz	650g	1lb 7oz
75g	3oz	675g	1½lb
100g	3 oz	700g	1lb 9oz
125g	4oz	750g	1lb 11oz
140g	4 oz	800g	1¾lb
150g	5oz	900g	2lb
165g	5 oz	1kg	2¼lb
175g	6oz	1.1kg	2½lb
200g	7oz	1.25kg	2¾lb
225g	8oz	1.35kg	3lb
250g	9oz	1.5kg	3lb 6oz
275g	10oz	1.8kg	4lb
300g	11oz	2kg	4½lb
350g	12oz	2.25kg	5lb
375g	13oz	2.5kg	5½lb
		2.75kg	6lb

LIQUID MEASURES

Metric	Imperial	Aus	US
25ml	1fl oz		
50ml	2fl oz	¼ cup	¼ cup
75ml	3fl oz		
100ml	3 fl oz		
120ml	4fl oz	½ cup	½ cup
150ml	5fl oz		
175ml	6fl oz	¾ cup	¾ cup
200ml	7fl oz		
250ml	8fl oz	1 cup	1 cup
300ml	10fl oz/½ pint	½ pint	1¼ cups
360ml	12fl oz		
400ml	14fl oz		
450ml	15fl oz	2 cups	2½ cups/1 pint
600ml	1 pint	1 pint	2 cups
750ml	1¼ pints		
900ml	1½ pints		
1 litre	1¾ pints	1¾ pints	1 quart
1.2 litres	2 pints		
1.4 litres	2½ pints		
1.5 litres	2½ pints		
1.7 litres	3 pints		
2 litres	3½ pints		
3 litres	5¼ pints		

UK-Australian tablespoon conversions

1 x UK or Australian teaspoon is 5ml

1 x UK tablespoon is 3 teaspoons/15ml

1 Australian tablespoon is 4 teaspoons/20ml

Acknowledgements

Special thanks to Susan Murray for her assistance with Chapter Two.

Karen Thomson:
There are so many people who've had a profound impact on my life. This book is a sum of all of those parts. To Steven Thomson, Kobus Visser, Deirdre Barnard Visser, Tiaan Visser, Jamie Thomson and Luke Thomson, for teaching me what unconditional love and acceptance is. For protecting and loving me.

To special people Emily Maguire, Gary Wright, Kerry Hammerton, Adam Pike, Brigid Kell, Jemima-Faye Goodall, Jo and Charlotte Ashworth, Amy Daniels, Lisa Sonn, Michele Riley, Bryan Teare, Rita Fernandes Venter and Farahnaaz Dyer. Also fitting that description are all the HELP Harmony Eating & Lifestyle Program, The Sugar Free Revolution Online, Banting 101 and Harmony Addictions Group staff and patients. You made this book possible.

My earth angel Val Valentini, you've had such an impact on my life. You helped fix broken wings and taught me to fly.

The fantastic team at Little, Brown, especially Duncan Proudfoot, Florence Partridge and Clive Hebard, thank you for giving *Sugar Free* a chance.

Dr Aseem Malhotra for leading this health revolution in the UK. You have the courage of a lion, fearlessly fighting for what is right. My admiration and respect for you is endless.

My superhero and mentor Prof. Tim Noakes. Your belief in my abilities has empowered me to climb mountains; your tenacity, wisdom and ability to stand in your truth and speak from the heart reminds me so much of my brilliant grandfather.

Emily Maguire:
My inspiration comes from all
of the health professionals and
researchers who have not given up.
They have continued their work
in the face of great adversity and
thanks to them, I and others like
me have been able to move away
from our conventional training.

Particular thanks go to
Professor Richard Feinman,
Dr Jeff Volek, Dr Steve Phinney,
and Dr Will Yancy from Duke
University, and above all to Dr Eric
Westman. He truly is one of the
pioneers within this field, not only
producing great research but also
working one on one with patients
to implement this way of life.

I also need to send a huge
thank you to my family and
friends who have always
supported me. Especially to my
parents, as without their support,
encouragement and belief in me
I really would not be where I am
today. And lastly, I have to say a
huge thank you to my soul sister,
Karen Thomson. You are truly
one of the most inspiring people
I know.

Index

Index of Recipes

CHAPTER FOURTEEN

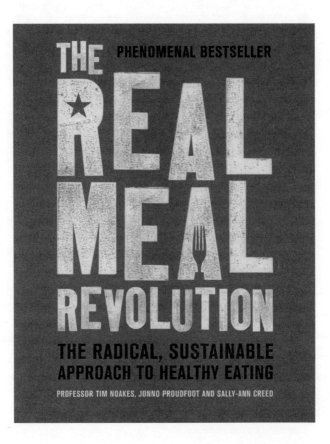

PHENOMENAL BESTSELLER

THE REAL MEAL REVOLUTION

THE RADICAL, SUSTAINABLE APPROACH TO HEALTHY EATING

PROFESSOR TIM NOAKES, JONNO PROUDFOOT AND SALLY-ANN CREED

The Real Meal Revolution

The Radical, Sustainable Approach to Healthy Eating
Prof Tim Noakes, Jonno Proudfoot and Sally-Ann Creed

Available to buy in ebook and paperback

We've been told for years that eating fat is bad for us, that it is a primary cause of high blood pressure, heart disease and obesity. *The Real Meal Revolution* debunks this lie and shows us the way back to restored health through eating what human beings are meant to eat.

The work of a scientist, a nutritionist and a chef, this phenomenal bestseller turns their extensive research and experience into a definitive eating guide and cookbook, packed with simple, delicious and beautifully photographed recipes, that will radically transform your health.
You will take control of not just your weight, but your overall health, too – through what you eat. And you can eat meat, seafood, eggs, cheese, butter, nuts ... often the first things to be prohibited or severely restricted on most diets. This is Banting, or Low-Carb, High-Fat (LCHF) eating, for a new generation, solidly underpinned by years of scientific research and by now incontrovertible evidence.

THE REAL MEAL REVOLUTION

SUPER FOOD FOR SUPERCHILDREN

DELICIOUS, LOW-SUGAR RECIPES FOR HEALTHY,
HAPPY FAMILIES, FROM TODDLERS TO TEENS

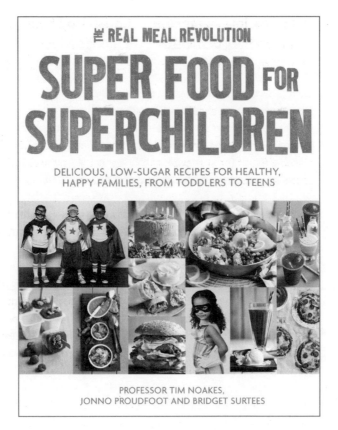

PROFESSOR TIM NOAKES,
JONNO PROUDFOOT AND BRIDGET SURTEES

Super Food for Superchildren

Delicious, low-sugar recipes for healthy, happy children, from toddlers to teens
Prof Tim Noakes, Jonno Proudfoot and Bridget Surtees

Available to buy in ebook and paperback

There is so much dietary advice out there, much of it conflicting, that it can be difficult for busy parents to make sense of it all. Medical doctor and sports scientist, Professor Tim Noakes, chef and long-distance swimmer, Jonno Proudfoot, and dietitian Bridget Surtees, a specialist in paediatric nutrition, cut through the clamour to provide clear, proven guidelines and simple, delicious recipes to feed your family well, inexpensively and without fuss.

Following their record-breaking success with *The Real Meal Revolution*, the Real Meal team set out to rethink the way we feed our children. The result, *Superfood for Superchildren*, challenges many ingrained dietary beliefs and advocates a real-food diet for children that is low in sugar and refined carbohydrates. Their advice is solidly underpinned by a critical, scientific interrogation of the children's food industry.

By combining the latest peer-reviewed scientific evidence with straightforward, mouthwatering recipes, most of them for the whole family, this book shows clearly how to provide your children with the best possible nutrition to help them to grow up healthy and happy.

THE
IMPRVEMENT
ZONE

Looking for life inspiration?

The Improvement Zone has it all, from **expert advice** on how to advance your **career**, improve your **relationships**, boost your **business**, revitalise your **health** or develop your **mind**. Whatever your goals, head to our website now.

www.improvementzone.co.uk

INSPIRATION ON THE MOVE

INSPIRATION DIRECT TO YOUR INBOX